Microvascular Reconstructive Surgery of the Face

Guest Editor

MARK K. WAX, MD, FACS, FRCS(C)

FACIAL PLASTIC SURGERY CLINICS OF NORTH AMERICA

www.facialplastic.theclinics.com

May 2009 • Volume 17 • Number 2

SAUNDERS an imprint of ELSEVIER, Inc.

W.B. SAUNDERS COMPANY
A Division of Elsevier Inc.

1600 John F. Kennedy Blvd., Suite 1800, Philadelphia, PA 19103-2899

http://www.theclinics.com

FACIAL PLASTIC SURGERY CLINICS OF NORTH AMERICA Volume 17, Number 2
May 2009 ISSN 1064-7406, ISBN 1-4377-0474-3, 978-1-4377-0474-7

Editor: Joanne Husovski
Developmental Editor: Donald Mumford

Facial Plastic Surgery Clinics of North America (ISSN 1064-7406) is published quarterly by Elsevier Inc., 360 Park Avenue South, New York, NY 10010-1710. Months of issue are February, May, August, and November. Business and Editorial Offices: 1600 John F. Kennedy Blvd., Suite 1800, Philadelphia, PA 19103-2899. Periodicals postage paid at New York, NY, and additional mailing offices. Subscription prices are $273.00 per year (US individuals), $428.00 per year (US institutions), $307.00 per year (Canadian individuals), $513.00 per year (Canadian institutions), $368.00 per year (foreign individuals), $513.00 per year (foreign institutions), $133.00 per year (US students), and $185.00 per year (foreign students). Foreign air speed delivery is included in all *Clinics* subscription prices. All prices are subject to change without notice. POSTMASTER: Send address changes to *Facial Plastic Surgery Clinics*, Elsevier Periodicals Customer Service, 11830 Westline Industrial Drive, St. Louis, MO 63146. **Customer service: 1-800-654-2452 (US and Canada); 1-314-453-7041 (outside US and Canada); Fax: 314-453-5170; E-mail: journalscustomerservice-usa@elsevier.com (for print support); journalsonlinesupport-usa@elsevier.com (for online support).**

Reprints. For copies of 100 or more of articles in this publication, please contact the Commercial Reprints Department, Elsevier Inc., 360 Park Avenue South, New York, NY 10010-1710. Tel.: 212-633-3812; Fax: 212-462-1935; E-mail: reprints@elsevier.com.

Facial Plastic Surgery Clinics of North America is covered in *MEDLINE/PubMed* (*Index Medicus*).

Printed and bound by CPI Group (UK) Ltd, Croydon, CR0 4YY

Transferred to Digital Print 2011

Contributors

CONSULTING EDITOR

J. REGAN THOMAS, MD
Lederer Professor and Chairman, Department
of Otolaryngology—Head and Neck Surgery,
University of Illinois at Chicago College of
Medicine, Chicago, Illinois

EDITORIAL BOARD

SHAN R. BAKER, MD
Professor and Chief, Section of Plastic
and Reconstructive Surgery, University
of Michigan, Ann Arbor, Michigan

ROBERT KELLMAN, MD
Professor and Chairman, Department
of Otolaryngology, State University of New
York Upstate Medical University, Syracuse,
New York

RUSSELL W.H. KRIDEL, MD
Clinical Associate Professor, Department of
Otolaryngology—Head and Neck Surgery,
Division of Facial Plastic Surgery, University of
Texas Health Science Center, Houston, Texas

STEPHEN W. PERKINS, MD
Private Practitioner, Perkins Facial Plastic
Surgery, Indianapolis, Indiana

ANTHONY P. SCLAFANI, MD, FACS
Director of Facial Plastic Surgery, The New
York Eye and Ear Infirmary, New York,
New York; and Professor of Otolaryngology—
Head and Neck Surgery, New York Medical
College, Valhalla, New York

GUEST EDITOR

MARK K. WAX, MD, FACS, FRCS(C)
Professor, Otolaryngolory-Head and Neck
Surgery; Professor, Oral and Maxillofacial
Surgery; Program Director, Otolaryngology-
Head and Neck Surgery; Director, Microvascular
Reconstruction; and Coordinator, Education
AAOHNS, Department of Otolaryngology-Head
& Neck Surgery, Oregon Health & Science
University, Portland, Oregon

AUTHORS

STEVEN B. CANNADY, MD
Microvascular Fellow, Oregon Health &
Science University, Portland, Oregon

DOUGLAS B. CHEPEHA, MD, FRCS(C)
Associate Professor, Department of
Otolaryngology; Director, Microvascular

Program; and Co-Chair, Research Committee, University of Michigan Medical Center, Ann Arbor, Michigan

TED A. COOK, MD
Professor, Oregon Health & Science University, Portland, Oregon

YADRANKO DUCIC, MD, FRCSC, FACS
Otolaryngology and Facial Plastic Surgery Associates, Fort Worth; Baylor Neuroscience Skull Base Center, Dallas/Fort Worth; The Center for Aesthetic Surgery, Colleyville; and University of Texas Southwestern Medical Center, Dallas, Texas

NEAL D. FUTRAN, MD, DMD
Professor and Chair, Department of Otolaryngology-Head and Neck Surgery; and Director of Head and Neck Surgery, University of Washington, Seattle, Washington

ERIC M. GENDEN, MD
Professor and Chairman, Department of Otolaryngology-Head and Neck Surgery; Professor, Institute for Immunobiology; and Director, Head and Neck Cancer Center, The Mount Sinai Medical Center, New York, New York

TAMER GHANEM, MD
Head and Neck Microvascular/Reconstructive Fellow, Department of Otolaryngology-Head and Neck Surgery, Oregon Health & Science University, Portland, Oregon

RALPH W. GILBERT, MD, FRCSC
Professor of Otolaryngology/Head and Neck Surgery, University of Toronto, Wharton Head and Neck Centre, Princess Margaret Hospital, Toronto, Ontario, Canada

TIM A. ISELI, MBBS, FRACS
Head and Neck Fellow, Division of Otolaryngology, Head & Neck Surgery, Department of Surgery, University of Alabama School of Medicine, Birmingham, Alabama

JEFFREY S. MOYER, MD, FACS
University of Michigan Medical Center, Ann Arbor, Michigan

MICHAEL J. ODELL, MD, FRCS(C)
Director, Head and Neck Oncology; Assistant Professor, Department of Otolaryngology-Head and Neck Surgery, Saint Louis University School of Medicine, St. Louis, Missouri

EUNICE E. PARK, MD, MPH
Department of Otolaryngology-Head and Neck Surgery, The Mount Sinai Medical Center, New York, New York

MARK E.P. PRINCE, MD, FRCS(C)
Assistant Professor, Otolaryngology/Head and Neck Surgery, University of Michigan Medical Center, Ann Arbor, Michigan

EBEN L. ROSENTHAL, MD
Associate Professor, Division of Otolaryngology, Head & Neck Surgery, Department of Surgery, University of Alabama School of Medicine, Birmingham, Alabama

MARK G. SHRIME, MD, FACS
Wharton Head and Neck Centre, Princess Margaret Hospital, Toronto, Ontario, Canada

THEODOROS N. TEKNOS, MD, FACS
Professor; Director, Division of Head and Neck Surgery; and David E. and Carole H. Schuller Chair in Head and Neck Oncologic Surgery, The Ohio State University Medical Center, Columbus, Ohio

MARK A. VARVARES, MD, FACS
Professor and Chairman, The Donald and Marlene Jerome Chair of Otolaryngology-Head and Neck Surgery, Department of Otolaryngology-Head and Neck Surgery; and Director, Saint Louis University Cancer Center, St. Louis, Missouri

MARK K. WAX, MD, FACS, FRCS(C)
Professor, Otolaryngolory-Head and Neck Surgery; Professor, Oral and Maxillofacial Surgery; Program Director, Otolaryngology-Head and Neck Surgery; Director, Microvascular Reconstruction; and Coordinator, Education AAOHNS, Department of Otolaryngology-Head & Neck Surgery, Oregon Health & Science University, Portland, Oregon

Contents

The scalp provides a relatively limited amount of excess tissue that can be used in reconstructing significant scalp defects, which arise most often from oncologic resection or traumatic loss. Scalp reconstruction encompasses a broad spectrum of flaps, grafts, and techniques that should be readily available to the facial plastic surgeon treating this patient population. Meticulous attention to detail, particularly in the planning and early postoperative periods, is associated with gratifying results in the majority of patients. This article presents defect analysis and discussion of reconstruction options, with figures of successful reconstructive surgeries.

The structures of the nose are arguably the most complex within the face to reconstitute when absent. Total nasal reconstruction has evolved to encompass advanced surgical techniques in an effort to achieve increasingly satisfactory cosmetic results while restoring nasal function that mimics the function of a patient's natural nose. In this article, the history of total nasal defects and their reconstruction, relevant nasal anatomy, etiologies of the defect, and the surgical approaches to reconstructing each of the three-layered structure of the nose (ie, nasal skin, cartilage/bone, and lining mucosa) are explored.

Reconstruction of extensive lip defects is a challenging task for reconstructive microsurgeons. This article reviews the goals of lip reconstruction after major ablative or traumatic lip losses and outlines the free flap options available to achieve these goals.

The maxilla and midface have an important aesthetic and functional role. Their reconstruction after surgical ablation is a complex problem. The historical development of reconstruction of the midface, classification systems of maxillary defects, and descriptions of reconstructive options are presented.

Extensive skin, paranasal, and skull base malignancies often invade the orbit necessitating the removal of the orbital contents to achieve local tumor control. Defects of this region often create a communication between the intracranial and extracranial contents that involves a large volume of skin, soft tissue, and bone. Local and regional tissue alone is rarely adequate to repair these defects. In contrast, free tissue transfer can provide vascularized skin, soft tissue, and bone that can reliably separate the extracranial and intracranial compartments and restore the bony and soft tissue architecture of the orbitomaxillary complex. This article summarizes the approach to orbitomaxillary reconstruction and discusses the use of free tissue transfer in the rehabilitation of this complex region.

Maxillofacial trauma caused by severe ballistic or avulsion injuries to the face creates complex composite defects. The essential difference between most blunt facial injuries and ballistic or avulsive facial injuries is the severity of the soft and hard tissue loss and damage. Application of modern principles of fracture management and wound care, however, allows restoration of the facial framework until a healthy tissue bed is achieved for definitive repair. Free tissue transfer has made it possible to bring well-vascularized bone and soft tissue into a hostile wound environment with excellent survival of the flap tissues. This has allowed for simultaneous reconstruction of the bony facial skeleton and the overlying soft tissue soon after injury.

Large periauricular and temporal bone defects most commonly follow resection of advanced nonmelanoma skin cancers. Reconstruction aims to cover the cutaneous defect and adjacent vital structures with the ability to heal in an irradiated field and withstand further treatment. Preferred reconstructions are class I, cervicofacial rotation or radial forearm free flap; class II, anterolateral thigh; and class II, rectus abominis free flap. Ancillary procedures, especially for associated facial paralysis, often are required. Although free flap reconstruction provides rapid wound healing, local and regional flaps are alternatives for patients unable to tolerate prolonged anesthesia and for use after recurrence or complications.

Parotidectomy is a widely performed procedure for various indications, including benign and malignant conditions. For malignant neoplasms of the parotid gland or metastatic disease, it may be performed in conjunction with cheek or temple skin resection, facial nerve sacrifice, or composite resection of a portion of the mandible. There are various options for reconstruction depending on the extent of resection. This article discusses various reconstructive options following parotidectomy and other ablative procedures that are often performed in conjunction. Reconstruction of parotidectomy defects associated with lateral temporal bone resection is discussed elsewhere in this issue.

Facial reconstruction poses a unique surgical challenge—restoring the aesthetic form and function of the face. Established techniques for reconstruction include skin grafts, local cutaneous tissue flaps, and free flap autografts. The anatomic complexity of the face renders it challenging, however, to obtain a successful cosmetic and functional result. The success of recent hand, knee joint, and larynx allotransplantation and advances in immunosuppressive regimens have pushed the technical frontiers of composite tissue transfer to include partial facial transplantation. This article reviews current techniques for reconstruction of facial defects, with a focus on the microsurgical, immunologic, and ethical considerations of facial allotransplantation.

Skin cancer arising in the head and neck is a common occurrence. Although the vast majority of these cancers can be treated with simple excision and local reconstruction there is a subset of patients who have massive tumors that require composite tissue resection. These patients are best reconstructed with free tissue transfer. Acceptable functional and cosmetic results can be expected. Long-term survival is excellent in patients who have negative margins.

Facial Plastic Surgery Clinics of North America

THE CLINICS ARE NOW AVAILABLE ONLINE!

Access your subscription at:
www.theclinics.com

Preface

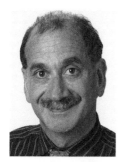

Mark K. Wax, MD, FACS, FRCS(C)
Guest Editor

Occasionally, the facial plastic reconstructive surgeon encounters a patient who has a composite defect that is not amenable to local tissue rearrangement. Whether the patient presents with such a large lesion that local tissues will not suffice for reconstructive purposes or the patient has been heavily pretreated by surgery or multiple surgical excisions with local flap reconstructions, tissue from outside of the head and neck area is required.

The advent of microvascular reconstructive surgery has allowed for composite soft tissue defects to be reconstructed with similar composite tissues from other parts of the body. Initially, microvascular free tissue transfer was used for reconstruction of oncologic and ablative defects encountered in the upper aerodigestive tract. The ability to decrease the infection rate, get patients out of the hospital more quickly, decrease the morbidity, and increase the potential rehabilitation quickly saw these surgical techniques become the preferred method of reconstruction. With this burgeoning experience of free tissue transfer came an ability to use this method of reconstruction in complex composite reconstruction of cutaneous defects.

The multitude of authors who have expertise in this area describe their experience in this issue of *Facial Plastic Surgery Clinics of North America* and demonstrate how some patients at the far end of the reconstructive spectrum can certainly be well rehabilitated and functionally reconstructed using free tissue transfer. The patient who has experienced severe composite tissue loss from trauma is able to be functionally reconstructed using a composite free tissue flap that often contains bone. Scalp and total nasal reconstruction are areas of increasing experience in this particular field.

Free tissue transfer is clearly not the reconstructive modality of choice for most patients who have defects of the head and neck area. Local tissue transfer still remains the most common method of reconstruction. In a select patient population, however, the multitude of composite tissues available for transfer certainly allows the facial plastic and reconstructive surgeon the ability to functionally and cosmetically reconstruct large defects.

Mark K. Wax, MD, FACS, FRCS(C)
Professor, Otolaryngology-Head and
Neck Surgery
Professor, Oral and Maxillofacial Surgery
Program Director, Otolaryngology-Head and
Neck Surgery
Director, Microvascular Reconstruction
Coordinator, Education AAOHNS
Oregon Health & Science University
3181 SW Sam Jackson Park Road PV-01
Portland, OR 97201

E-mail address:
waxm@ohsu.edu

Facial Plast Surg Clin N Am 17 (2009) ix
doi:10.1016/j.fsc.2009.01.010

facialplastic.theclinics.com

Reconstruction of the Scalp

Yadranko Ducic, MD, FRCSC, FACS[a,b,c,d,*]

KEYWORDS

• Scalp • Reconstruction • Free flaps • Tissue expander

The scalp represents the thick, durable covering that provides protection for the vital underlying calvarium and brain, serving as the first and likely most important barrier. It is composed of hair-bearing (temporal, parietal and occipital) and non–hair-bearing skin (frontal), underlying occipitofrontalis muscle (connected by the galea aponeurotica) gliding over a thin sheet of nourishing pericranium (**Fig. 1**). Most scalp avulsions occur within this loose areolar tissue plane, often leaving the pericranium nonviolated and facilitating reconstruction. The skin of the scalp is the thickest in the body, varying from 3 to 8 mm in depth. The neurovascular structures supplying the scalp traverse through the deep subcutaneous tissues overlying the galea aponeurotica. There is an extensive collateral network of vessels providing the scalp with its blood supply (**Fig. 2**), which enables the creation of a number of reliable random pattern flaps to be raised successfully. The supraorbital and supratrochlear vessels provide the anterior contribution to this network, joining the posterior auricular branch from the external carotid artery and the superficial temporal superficial artery laterally and the occipital arteries posteriorly. Scalp innervation is provided by the trigeminal nerve and by branches of the cervical plexus.

The skull itself is composed of inner and outer tables that are variable in thickness between the different parts of the skull; between individuals; and, that change as one progresses from infancy through adulthood. The calvarium is somewhat malleable in children, which is clinically relevant in terms of providing a source of easily contoured grafts used in reconstructive surgery. Conversely, the skull of the elderly is more brittle and less amenable to alteration of its basic original shape. However, in adults, the overlying scalp is more pliable and occasionally slightly redundant as compared with the scalps of young children. At all ages, the scalp provides a relatively limited amount of excess tissue that can be used in reconstructing significant scalp defects, which arise most often from oncologic resection or traumatic loss.

In 1696, Belloste described perforating the bare skull to allow for granulation tissue formation and to promote subsequent epithelaization.[1] In the late 1800s, Netolitzky subsequently introduced skin graft placement on the granulation tissue bed to expedite the healing process.[2] Kazanjian and others espoused the use of local flaps.[3,4] The area providing the most scalp mobility is in the region overlying the temporal fossa, making this region an ideal scalp flap donor area. Conversely, the lateral frontal region provides relatively little extra mobility, rendering the need for relatively large flaps to be elevated to close even small defects in this region. Radovan popularized tissue expansion of the scalp, enabling recruitment of more hair bearing adjacent scalp.[5] Extensive defects or avulsive injuries of the scalp have been successfully treated for a number of years with microsurgical reattachment and free tissue transfer.[6–10]

DEFECT ANALYSIS

There are many considerations when formulating a treatment plan for a given patient with a scalp

[a] Otolaryngology and Facial Plastic Surgery Associates, Fort Worth, TX, USA
[b] Baylor Neuroscience Skull Base Center, Dallas/Fort Worth, TX, USA
[c] The Center for Aesthetic Surgery, Colleyville, TX, USA
[d] University of Texas Southwestern Medical Center, Dallas, TX, USA
* Otolaryngology and Facial Plastic Surgery Associates, 923 Pennsylvania Avenue Suite 100, Fort Worth, TX 76104.
E-mail address: yducic@sbcglobal.net

Facial Plast Surg Clin N Am 17 (2009) 177–187
doi:10.1016/j.fsc.2009.01.001

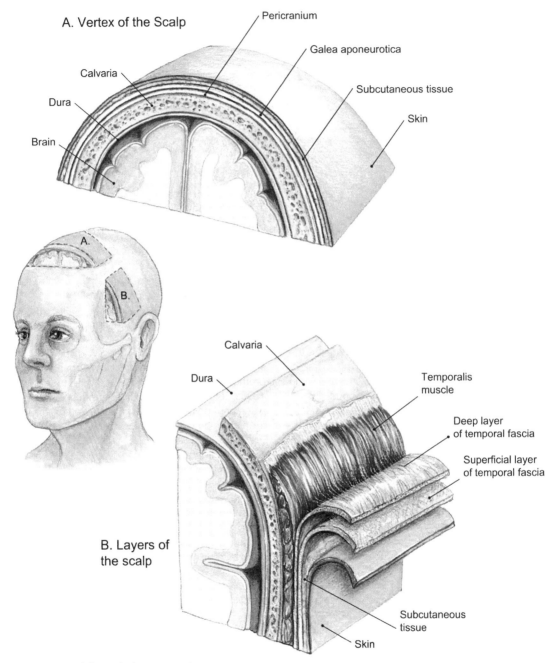

Fig. 1. Layers of the scalp in cross section.

defect. Patient expectations and comorbid conditions need to be taken into account. Patient tolerance for certain procedures may limit their utility—particularly in the case of prolonged tissue expansion. Far and away the best tissue for replacement of lost scalp is adjacent scalp tissue. Particular attention needs to be paid to the present hair distribution and its anticipated future. Small areas of alopecia or hairless flap may be covered by hair transplantation. Hair transplantation is not feasible in large flap reconstruction and it is often not reliably successful in patients undergoing perioperative radiation therapy. Local flap reconstruction in this latter group of patients is more difficult due to regional fibrosis and diminished blood supply.[11] In this group of patients, there is a need for broader based, larger breadth local "scalping" flaps and free tissue transfer.[12,13]

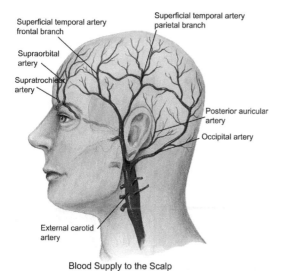

Superficial temporal artery
frontal branch

Superficial temporal artery
parietal branch

Supraorbital
artery

Supratrochlear
artery

Posterior auricular
artery

Occipital artery

External carotid
artery

Blood Supply to the Scalp

Fig. 2. Major vascular supply to the scalp that is used when designing scalp flaps.

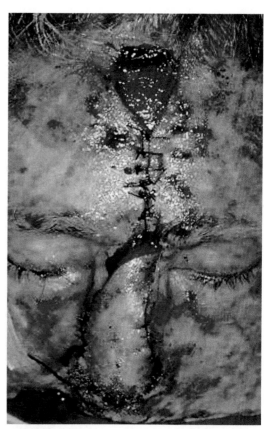

Fig. 4. Intraoperative view of patient following inset of forehead flap with persistent open wound forehead. Note that the underlying pericranium is intact.

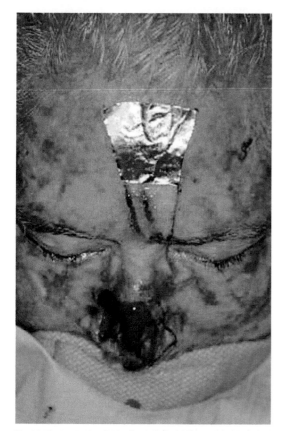

Fig. 3. Intraoperative view of patient undergoing nasal reconstruction with a forehead flap following Moh's excision of basal cell carcinoma.

RECONSTRUCTIVE OPTIONS
Wound Care and Healing by Secondary Intention

The simplest form of reconstruction is nonsurgical. Simple, good, meticulous and prolonged wound care has the ability to heal relatively large scalp defects surprisingly well. Healing by secondary intention works best in non–hair-bearing areas of the scalp or in relatively follicle-challenged areas of age related alopecia. It does cause some distortion of the immediately surrounding areas and should be used with caution in the periorbital region because of potential brow distortion. The scars themselves tend to be atrophic and contain telangiectasias, which may be visually distracting.[14] Nevertheless, the final aesthetic result is reasonable. If there is overlying pericranium, the healing process may be completed in as little as 3 weeks for defects less than 2 cm and in as long as 2 to 3 months for larger defects. If there is no pericranial covering to the scalp, then consideration of burring the outer table to promote granulation tissue formation and then allowing for secondary intention healing to take place is reasonable. Prolonged wound care with hydration-promoting antibiotic-impregnated gauze dressing is required in all of these patients. Prevention of dessication is of paramount importance (**Figs. 3–6**).

Skin Grafting for Scalp Defects

In 1908, Robinson described successful skin grafting when these grafts were applied directly to an intact underlying pericranium.[15] Traditionally, skin grafts have not done well when placed directly on exposed calvarium without first having had a granulation tissue bed beneath. The major difficulty with this has been lack of traction between the graft and underlying bare skull. Micromotion or macromotion will not allow for graft revascularization in time to save it from invariable dessication and loss. Skin grafts may be used for temporary coverage, minimizing wound care issues while preparing the scalp for definitive reconstruction, as during prolonged tissue expansion. When used, skin grafts should be

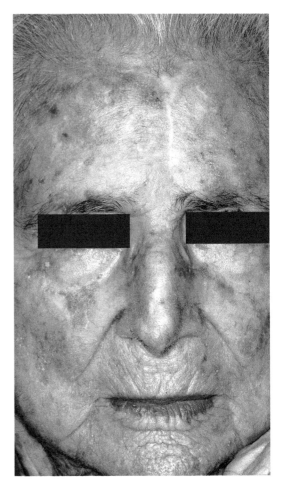

Fig. 6. Final postoperative result. Note well-healed forehead wound with thin scar.

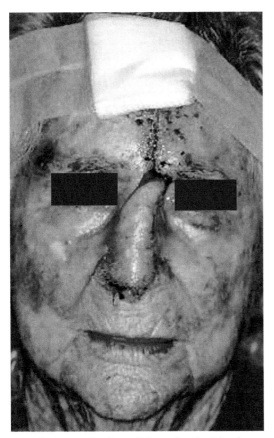

Fig. 5. Postoperative frontal view of patient (as shown in **Figs. 1–4**) with dressing in position.

unmeshed to give the best possible appearance. (**Figs. 7–9**).

Primary coverage with a skin graft, followed by serial excision, is an option for patients not desiring tissue expansion and wanting to maintain a relatively normal hair distribution. Skin grafts may also be used to provide coverage for free muscle flaps to decrease the flap bulk that would otherwise be seen in patients if the muscle and full thickness skin were transplanted as a single unit as in the case of latissimus or rectus free flaps (**Fig. 10**).

Primary Closure of Scalp Wounds and Rapid Intraoperative Tissue Expansion

Temporal scalp defects or low central frontal scalp defects, especially in elderly patients, may often be closed by simple, wide undermining in a subgaleal plane. Galeal incisions placed parallel to the incision may help recruit 1 to 1.5 cm of tissue to

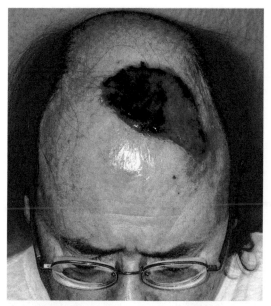

Fig. 7. Preoperative view of patient with history of chronic nonhealing wound for over 2 years following excision of basal cell carcinoma.

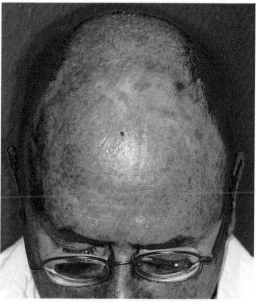

Fig. 9. Long-term (1 year) result demonstrating well-healed skin graft with reasonable color match to surrounding tissue. Some atrophic changes, as seen here, are to be expected. This result is adequate in an individual with advanced alopecia as in this patient.

help decrease wound tension during closure. For small defects up to 3 cm in nonradiated patients, undermining in a subcutaneous tissue plane may allow for more recruitment of skin into the defect. This strategy is at the expense of tensile strength and vascularity, limiting its use in larger defects or for radiated individuals.

Rapid intraoperative tissue expansion (RITE) produces no additional collagen formation, instead working on the principle of mechanical creep.[16] With RITE, there is deformation of the three-dimensional structure of the collagen fibrils,

which allows for increased length of these fibrils, recruiting additional adjacent tissue. An expanded Foley catheter balloon may be inflated and maintained for at least 5 minutes. It works best if it is placed adjacent to the defect and if mechanical tension is maintained along the wound edges with either sutures or clamps during the expansion process. This is primarily a technique that will help reduce tension across the closure line in defects that are closed with local or regional flaps and where the skin closure is taut.

Tissue Expansion

Tissue expansion over a prolonged period of time results in the phenomenon of biologic creep. As opposed to mechanical creep with simple distortion of the three-dimensional collagen fibrils, with biologic creep there is actually deposition of new collagen over time. By necessity, scalp tissue expansion takes a prolonged period of time, perhaps even months for large defects. Approximately 50% of the scalp can be reconstructed with extended periods of tissue expansion.[17] It is important to provide for safe coverage of the defect during the time of expansion. This need is often facilitated by skin graft placement at the time of expander insertion.

There are various shapes and sizes of expanders that are commercially available

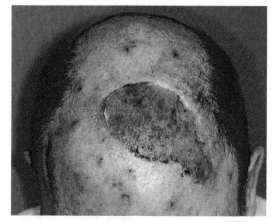

Fig. 8. Early postoperative result following skin graft placement following excision of the nonhealing wound to the level of the calvarium.

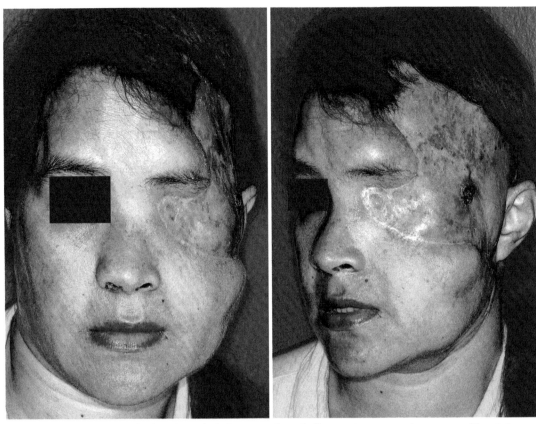

Fig. 10. Well-healed skin graft placed on a latissimus muscle–only flap used to cover a large area of frontotemporal scalp that had undergone post radiation soft tissue necrosis.

(Fig. 11). In general, the largest expander possible should be chosen and it should be placed in a subgaleal plane. The shape of the expander also affects the amount of tissue gained in the expansion process, with more biologic creep noted as one goes from round to crescent-shaped to rectangle-shaped expanders.[18] Also, it is best to choose a single large expander than multiple smaller ones because this results in maximal gain of tissue per volume of expansion. In laterally placed defects, a central adjacent large expander works well. However, in more centrally placed

Fig. 11. Commonly used rectangular tissue expander with attached injection port is most efficient for scalp reconstruction. Size selection depends on defect dimensions and should be carefully planned.

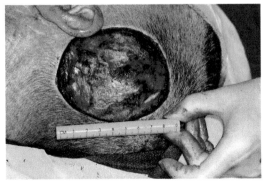

Fig. 12. Surgical defect left following excision of neglected massive melanoma of postauricular scalp.

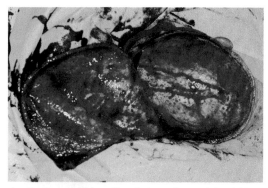

Fig. 13. Transposition flap being elevated in patient who is shown in Fig. 10.

defects, multiple expanders placed lateral to the defect tend to work more effectively. The expander is typically inserted and inflated to 10% to 20% of its volume at insertion, which eliminates any dead space and the need for drain insertion postoperatively. Tissue expansion is begun after 2 weeks and continued until the desired tissue gain has been achieved. One can estimate the amount of tissue gained with expansion by subtracting the base of the expander from the length over top of the expander and adding an extra 20% to 25% to counteract the recoil that is seen

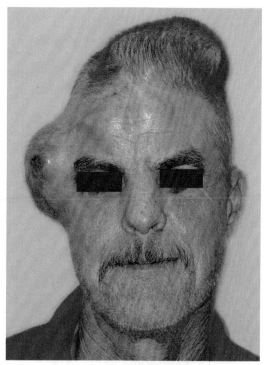

Fig. 15. Tissue expanders in position and maximally inflated.

during flap advancement. The ideal flap is raised as an advancement type flap along the sides of the implant.

After the desired amount of flap gain has been achieved, an additional 2 weeks should be allowed before flap harvest to allow for the biologic creep achieved by the last round of expansion. Infectious complications with tissue expanders are uncommon and they can usually be salvaged with antibiotics but may require implant replacement if the infection progresses. Implant exposure may occur. If it occurs late in the expansion process, the implant should be maintained in its expanded state, antibiotic-impregnated gauze covering of the exposed area, and antibiotic coverage maintained for two weeks following exposure to take advantage of the tissue gain maximally.

Meticulous planning is required when placing tissue expanders. If at all possible, one should aim to recreate or improve the existing hair distribution. There is some controversy about skin incision placement relative to the hair follicles. Incisions that cut across the hair follicles because of perpendicular placement will result in a softer appearance but may result in localized alopecia, whereas incisions placed parallel to the follicles may be more discernible—especially when the

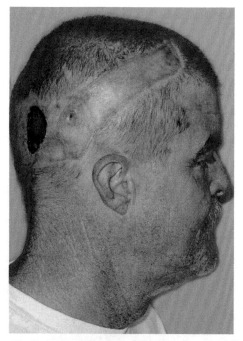

Fig. 14. Postoperative view following rotation flap coverage of postauricular scalp wound and skin graft application to donor site.

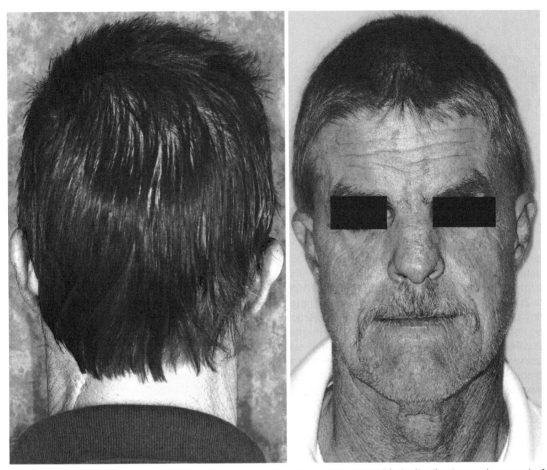

Fig. 16. Postoperative views of patient who is shown in **Figs. 10–13**. Note normal hair distribution and removal of the skin grafted area.

hair is wet—but will result in the disruption of fewer hair follicles and thus decrease the risk of alopecia **(Figs. 12–16)**.[19]

Local Flap Reconstruction: Advancement, Rotation and Transposition

Designing local flaps for scalp reconstruction is based on same basic principles as in other parts of the body except that the flaps are generally longer for a given size defect because of the relatively inelastic nature of the scalp.[20] For small defects of generally less than 3 cm in the forehead and temple regions and even smaller in the parieto-occipital scalp, simple wide undermining and advancement flap closure is feasible with or without RITE to decrease wound closure tension. Most other flaps are either rotation or transposition. Ideally, one should design both of these latter two flaps with a named vascular pedicle entering its base. In addition, sufficient consideration must be given to maintenance of as normal

a hairline and hair distribution pattern as possible. Multiple rotation flaps may be designed particularly in vertex defects.[4] Generally, transposition flaps should be transposed from the posterior donor region to an anterior recipient region to allow for hairline maintenance in most individuals.

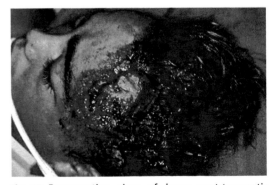

Fig. 17. Preoperative view of large post-traumatic wound of frontotemporal scalp.

If a patient has severe alopecia and a posterior scalp defect, it is acceptable to go in the reverse direction. Rotational flaps, and to a lesser extent, transposition flaps, result in significant standing cutaneous cones. These should be trimmed only very conservatively—and never in the region of the blood inflow tract—to decrease the risk of flap compromise. They will universally settle over a couple of months. If undesirable fullness is noted long-term, it is easily and safely dealt with secondarily after complete healing and peripheral neovascularization has occurred (**Figs. 17–19**).

Microvascular Free Tissue Transfer Reconstruction of the Scalp

Free tissue transfer of the scalp was first described by Mclean in 1972 when he covered a scalp wound with omentum.[21] Broad excision of many scalp malignancies results in removal of underlying periosteum as well, leaving the subsequent wound unsuitable for skin grafting. Defects of more than half of the forehead in patients with an intact hairline are well reconstructed with radial forearm free flaps because scalp flaps would result in movement of hair follicles into a hairless

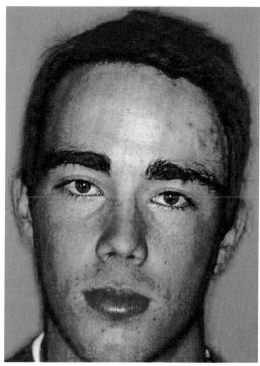

Fig. 19. Postoperative frontal view demonstrating adequate hairline distribution and relatively hidden scars.

region. Scalp flaps are still a good option in patients with significant alopecia. Latissimus and rectus free flaps, muscle only or with overlying skin in thin individuals, represent a nice reconstructive in the patient with massive soft tissue loss. When there is nonviable bone (eg, osteitis) secondary to radiation therapy beneath the area of marginal or absent scalp, free flap coverage should be considered. Free flaps appear to be able to tolerate therapeutic doses of radiation well (**Fig. 20**).[22]

The aforementioned free flaps all have reasonable length vessels that can reach the superficial temporal vessels and, if these are unavailable, performing anastomosis directly in the neck to branches of the external carotid artery.[23] The author of this article does not use the occipital vessels because postoperative positioning issues renders them at continued risk of compression. Postoperative positioning is very important in preventing loss of the flap or portions thereof. In a 10-year review of free tissue transfer reconstruction of scalp defects at MD Anderson, a complication rate of 59% was noted in the study group.[12] Most of these complications represented issues with delayed wound healing, particularly in larger flaps. This author has employed halos in large posterior reconstructions to decrease the risk of early

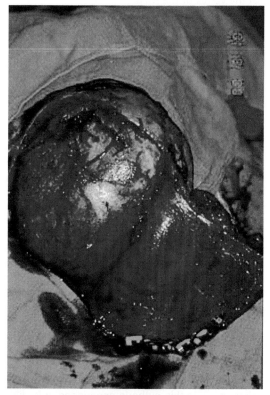

Fig. 18. Rotation scalping flap raised and ready for inset. Design was made to optimize frontotemporal hairline.

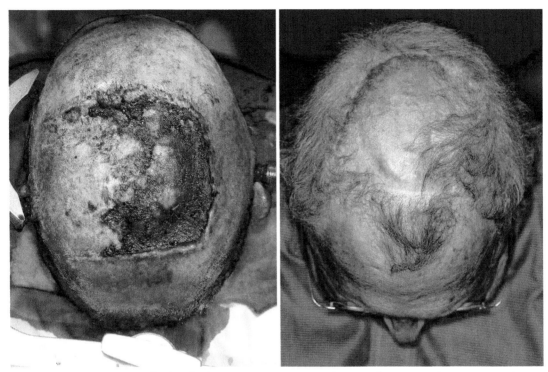

Fig. 20. Preoperative view (*left photo*) of patient status post craniectomy for metastatic prostate carcinoma. Neurosurgical flap design resulted in unfortunate loss of access flap. Postoperative view (*right photo*) demonstrating well healed radial forearm free flap reconstructionof the vertex of the scalp.

postoperative compression from patient positioning (see **Fig. 20**).

Skullbase Microvascular Reconstruction with Anastomosis at the Level of the Scalp

The majority of patients undergoing skullbase extirpative procedures do not require free tissue transfer reconstruction. There is a small subset of patients in which it is invaluable, consisting of the multiply-operated-on patient who has had loss of the pericranium as a potential flap and who has a large, often post-traumatic bony defect of the base of skull and ongoing cerebrospinal fluid leak. In such cases, a radial forearm fascial flap or a rectus muscle flap secured across the skull base from an intracranial approach is valuable. A key hole is made in the calvarium ipsilateral to the anastomosis that is performed in the temporal region of the scalp.[24] The edges of these flaps need to be inset with transosseous tunnels to prevent flap prolapsed inferiorly.

Adjunctive Techniques

Hair transplantation is often beneficial for areas of alopecia, reconstitution of the anterior hairline, or scar camouflage. Standard single and multifollicle grafts may be used with success.

When oncologic resection results in loss of scalp and underlying calvarium, there are a number of options for reconstruction. Autografts using rib, split calvarium, or iliac crest represent good alternatives and they may be preferable in the patient who has had osteitis or radiation therapy because of the increased risk of infection of alloplasts in these cases.[12] In fact, it may not be necessary to reconstruct the calvarium at all if there has been good free tissue transfer scalp coverage of the defect—even in patients who have a history of persistent scalp osteomyelitis.[13] In cases of chronic osteomyelitis of the calvarium arising as a sequala of either prior radiation therapy or a non-healing wound resulting from previous failed reconstruction or trauma, it is necessary to excise the necrotic bone. Systemic antibiotic therapy is clearly not going to penetrate necrotic nonvascularized bone or bone sequestra.[25] Free-tissue transfer can also incorporate bone stock as a single source for coverage of both scalp and calvarium.[26] In this author's experience, it is difficult to orient the bone graft portion of the flap to provide for an ideal bony reconstruction because of the relatively fixed orientation of the bone in relation to the pedicle and planned anastomosis. It is likely best used infrequently and with only small osseous defects. Alloplastic reconstruction of the skull, including methylmethacrylate, titanium mesh, hydroxyapatite cement, and CT-generated prefabricated acrylic, all represent viable options for replacement of the calvarium and protection of the underlying brain.[27,28]

SUMMARY

Scalp reconstruction encompasses a broad spectrum of flaps, grafts, and techniques that should be readily available to the facial plastic surgeon treating this patient population. Meticulous attention to detail, particularly in the planning and early postoperative periods, will be associated with gratifying results in the majority of patients.

REFERENCES

1. Strayer LM. Augustin Belloste and the treatment of avulsion of the scalp. N Engl J Med 1939;220:901–4.
2. Netolitzky J. Zur Kasuistik der Hauttranplantation. Wien Med Wochenschr 1871;21:820–2.
3. Kazanjian VH. Repair of partial losses of the scalp. Plast Reconstr Surg 1953;12:325–7.
4. Orticochea M. New three flap reconstruction technique. Br J Plast Surg 1971;24:184–7.
5. Radovan C. Tissue expansion in soft tissue reconstruction. Plast Reconstr Surg 1984;74:482–6.
6. Chicarelli ZN, Ariyan S, Cuono CB. Single stage repair of complex scalp and cranial defects with the radial forearm free flap. Plast Reconstr Surg 1986;77:577–85.
7. Miller GD, Anstee EJ, Snell JA. Successful replanatation of an avulsed scalp by microvascular anastomosis. Plast Reconstr Surg 1976;58:133–5.
8. Ionnides C, Fossion E, Mcgrouther AD. Reconstruction for large defects of the scalp and cranium. J Craniomaxillofac Surg 1999;27:145–50.
9. Lutz BS, Wei FC, Chen HC. Reconstruction of scalp defects with free flaps in 30 cases. Br J Plast Surg 1998;51:186–91.
10. Pennington DG, Stern HS, Lee KK. Free flap reconstruction of large defects of the scalp and calvarium. Plast Reconstr Surg 1989;84:655–71.
11. Oishi SN, Luce EA. The difficult scalp and skull wound. Clin Plast Surg 1995;22:51–7.
12. Hussussian CJ, Reece GP. Microsurgical scalp reconstruction in the patient with cancer. Plast Reconstr Surg 2002;109:1828–34.
13. Boeckx WD, van der Hulst RRWJ, Nanhekhan LV, et al. The role of free flaps in the treatment of persistent scalp osteomyelitis. Neurosurgery 2006;1:64–7.
14. Ranham GH. Reconstruction issues after Mohs surgery. Facial Plast Surg Clin North Am 1998;6:379–84.
15. Robinson EF. Total avulsion of the scalp. Surg Gynecol Obstet 1908;7:663–4.
16. Shapiro AL, Hochman M, Thomas JR, et al. Effects of intraoperative tissue expansion and skin flaps on wound closing tension. Arch Otolaryngol Head Neck Surg 1996;122:1107–10.
17. MAnders ER, Schenden MJ, Furrey JA, et al. Skin expansion to eliminate large scalp defects. Plast Reconstr Surg 1984;74:493–6.
18. Van Rappard JH, Molenaar J, van Doorn D, et al. Surface area increase in tissue expansion. Plast Reconstr Surg 1988;82:833–6.
19. Camirand A, Doucet J. A comparison between parallel hairline incisions and perpendicular incisions when performing a facelift. Plast Reconstr Surg 1995;99:10–4.
20. Ahuja RB. Geometric considerations in the design of rotational flaps in the scalp and forehead regions. Plast Reconstr Surg 1988;81:900–5.
21. Mclean DH, Buncke HJ. Autotransplant of omentum to a large scalp defect with microsurgical revascularization. Plast Reconstr Surg 1972;49:268–70.
22. Foote RL, Olsen KD, Meland NB, et al. Tumor ablative surgery, microvascular free tissue reconstruction, and postoperative radiation therapy for advanced head and neck cancer. Mayo Clin Proc 1994;69:122–6.
23. Hierner R, van Loon J, Goffin J, et al. Free latissimus dorsi flap transfer for subtotal scalp and cranium defect reconstruction: report of 7 cases. Microsurgery 2007;27:425–8.
24. Hansen SL, Foster RD, Dosanj AS, et al. Superficial temporal artery and vein as recipient vessels for facial and microsurgical reconstruction. Plast Reconstr Surg 2007;120:1879–84.
25. Ducic Y. Management of osteomyelitis of the anterior skull base and craniovertebral junction. Otolaryngol Head Neck Surg 2003;128:39–42.
26. Serra MP, Longhi P, Carminati M, et al. Microsurgical scalp and skull reconstruction using a combined flap composed of serratus anterior myo-osseous flap and latissimus dorsi myocutaneous flap. J Plast Reconstr Aesthet Surg 2007;60:1158–61.
27. Ducic Y. Titanium mesh and hydroxyapatite cement cranioplasty: a report of 20 cases. J Oral Maxillofac Surg 2002;60:272–6.
28. Verret DJ, Ducic Y, Oxford L, et al. Hydroxapatite cement in craniofacial reconstruction. Otolaryngol Head Neck Surg 2005;133:897–9.

The Total Nasal Defect and Reconstruction

Steven B. Cannady, MD, Ted A. Cook, MD,
Mark K. Wax, MD, FACS, FRCS(C)*

KEYWORDS

- Total nasal defect • Nasal reconstruction
- Nose amputation • Nose anatomic structure
- Forehead flap • Nasal surgical techniques

The nose is conspicuously located at the center of the face and therefore represents a crucial aesthetic focus to the observer and individual – a fact that imparted the legacy of rhinokopia (amputation of the nose) as a punishment in both Eastern and Western traditions.[1,2] Loss of a portion or the entirety of the nose greatly affects the perceived beauty of an individual and results in potentially catastrophic social limitations because of the public and private implications of arhinia. The structures of the nose are arguably the most complex within the face to reconstitute when absent, a fact which complicates nasal reconstruction. Complex three-dimensional architecture, multilayer construct, and functional importance underscore the difficulties associated with rebuilding nasal defects. Subtotal and partial defects of the nose allow the surgeon to employ techniques that rely on adjacent tissue transfer with acceptable cosmetic results.[3,4] However, the total nasal defect (Fig. 1), defined as "a bilateral through-and-through loss of nasal skin, cartilage/bone, and lining mucosa", beckons the reconstructive surgeon to utilize combinations of advanced locoregional soft tissue flaps, free cartilage or bone, and/or microvascular free tissue transfer to rehabilitate form and function.[5,6] Rooted in the surgical tradition of Indian rhinoplasty, total nasal reconstruction has evolved to encompass advanced surgical techniques in an effort to achieve increasingly satisfactory cosmetic results while restoring nasal function. In this article, the history of total nasal defects and their reconstruction, relevant nasal anatomy, etiologies of the defect, and the surgical approaches to reconstructing each of the three-layered structure of the nose are explored.

HISTORY OF TOTAL NASAL DEFECT AND RECONSTRUCTION

Most treatises on the surgical history of rhinoplasty and nasal reconstruction recognize an Indian work from the sixth century BC by Sushruta entitled *Samhita* as the origin of nasal reconstruction.[1,2] However, as illustrated by two recent reviews on the subject by Whitaker and colleagues[1] and Yalamanchili and colleagues,[2] nasal reconstructive techniques were probably devised much earlier and passed on by oral tradition among the potter classes of India beginning in 1500 BC.[2] In addition, writings on the treatment of nasal injuries date back to 3000 BC in the *Edwin Smith Surgical Papyrus*, as well as to Hippocrates' *Mochlicon*.[1]

The emergence of total nasal reconstructive technique is forever linked to the practice of nasal amputation and mutilation. The practice of rhinokopia was used as punishment for a variety of crimes, both social and moral, to permanently disfigure the offender and ultimately render them a labeled social outcast. The penalty was most often applied for thievery or adultery, for shaming the conquered of war, or for stigmatizing victims as in the case of deposed emperors.[2]

Perhaps the most impressive text on ancient nasal reconstruction, Suchruta's *Samhita* stands apart because of its depth in description and enduring techniques. Along with descriptions

Department of Otolaryngology-Head & Neck Surgery, Oregon Health & Science University, Physicians Pavilion 2nd floor, 3181 SW Sam Jackson Park Rd PV-01, Portland, OR 97239-3098, USA
* Corresponding author.
E-mail address: waxm@ohsu.edu (M.K. Wax).

Facial Plast Surg Clin N Am 17 (2009) 189–201
doi:10.1016/j.fsc.2009.01.002

facialplastic.theclinics.com

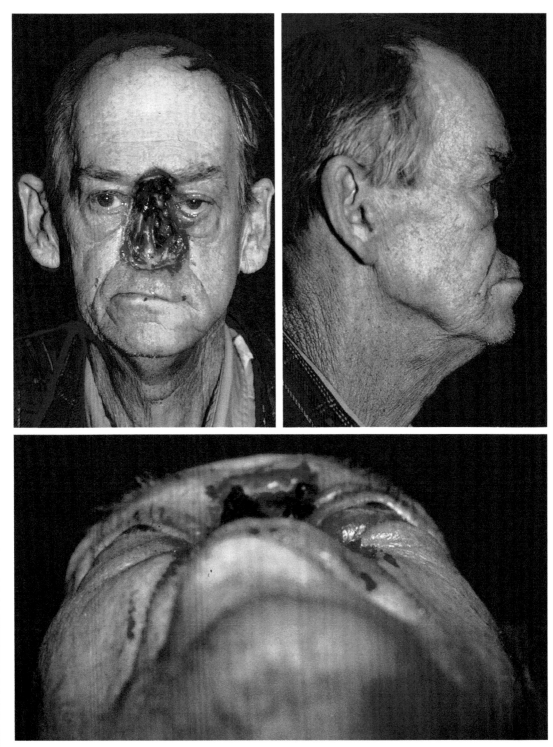

Fig. 1. The total nasal defect.

outlining surgical instrumentation, the need for individualized surgical planning with a leaf as a template, and meticulous suture technique and tissue opposition, Suchruta is credited with describing the first pedicled flap: the cheek advancement flap. The development of the paramedian forehead flap occurred later and is not well dated because of its practice by potter castes that passed the information via oral tradition rather than written text.[2]

Despite the long history of nasal reconstruction in India, the pedicled flap concept of total nasal reconstruction did not reach the West until much later, in the 1500s, when trade patterns exposed the techniques to Western surgeons. According to Yalamanchili's review, Indian techniques were passed to the West after they first penetrated Arabia and Persia and were translated to Latin around the seventh century. Next, Sicilians learned the techniques when the island served as a major Mediterranean trade center linking the East to the West in the thirteenth century. Modifications of the Indian technique were popularized by Tagliacozzi, a professor of anatomy at Bologna, who is credited with describing the "Italian method" in 1597, which involved a staged-arm flap to transfer viable skin to the nose. The Western world did not learn of the forehead flap until 1794 when a written description and illustration was submitted for publication in *Gentlemen's Magazine* in London.[2] European surgeons utilized cadaveric dissection to evaluate the techniques and allow for cautious adoption throughout the nineteenth century. The first American description was by John Mason Warren in 1834.[2]

Twentieth century modifications of the forehead flap have served to extend available tissue into the hairline, base the flap on unilateral supratrochlear vessels, and alter the orientation of the flap. The modern American use of the paramedian forehead flap was popularized by Kazanjian in 1946.[7] Subsequently, surgeons also have begun to recognize that the forehead flap represents a covering for the nose, but does not serve to reconstruct the structural support, or lining of the nose.[5,8–12] Changes in etiology of total nasal defects have sparked debates about treatments for the underlying causes and timing of reconstruction,[13,14] yet rhinectomy continues to be a viable surgical option for large skin cancers, and reconstruction of traumatic or systemic causes of the defect. Therefore, continued refinement and exploration of optimal timing and techniques for total nasal reconstruction promise new chapters in the long history outlined above.

RELEVANT ANATOMY AND FUNCTION OF THE NOSE

The face is divided into aesthetic subunits of which the nose is the most central. The nose is further divided into nine nasal subunits consisting of the lobule, dorsum, paired sidewalls, paired ala, paired soft tissue triangles, and the columella. Each subunit has a unique shape and concavity

or convexity that makes it distinctive to the eye and delineates it from the other subunits.[15,16] Although more important to partial nasal reconstructions, the subunit principle may apply to near-total defects in which it may be more cosmetic to sacrifice additional nasal skin to complete a subunit defect.[17,18]

Nasal skin varies in its thickness and sebaceous gland distribution with thick sebaceous skin overlying the lobule and alae, giving way to thinner less glandular skin over the dorsum, sidewalls, soft tissue triangles, and columella. In addition, each subunit has unique intranasal lining that warrants consideration. Skin lines the lobule, soft tissue triangles, and ala, whereas the columella is lined with the membranous skin that also lines the septum. The lining from the pyriform aperture and posterior becomes ciliated pseudostratified columnar epithelium and lines the dorsum and sidewalls; it is this portion of nasal lining that functions in secretion of mucous, trapping and transport of inhaled particles, and humidification and temperature control of the inhaled air. Ideally the reconstructive surgeon would replace missing structures with like ones; however, the nose is venerated with such intricate detail in shape, thickness, and function that it is often impossible to recreate the subunits of a nose following total rhinectomy.[17,18]

There is a rich anastamotic network of vessels to the overlying skin, to lining skin and to the mucosa of the nose. Although the vascular redundancy of the nose affords multiple local options for reconstruction, these options become more limited as defects approach total. However, local flaps are of utility in many cases and therefore the vascular supply in the region is important to review. Branches from the internal carotid (the anterior and posterior ethmoid arteries from the ophthalmic artery) and the external carotid (sphenopalatine, greater palatine, superior labial, and angular arteries) supply the nose. The external blood supply is chiefly derived from the facial artery, which is renamed the angular artery as it approaches the nasal ala. The dorsal aspect of the nose receives these branches and others from the internal maxillary artery (as the infraorbital arteries) and ophthalmic arteries. The blood supply to the nasal lining is via branches of the anterior and posterior ethmoid arteries; these vessels form anastamoses with the superior labial artery and greater palatine artery, respectively. Veins to the external and internal nose follow arterial patterns.[19]

The sensory innervation to the external and internal nasal lining is derived from the both the ophthalmic and maxillary divisions of the trigeminal nerve and includes the nasocilliary nerve (skin and mucous membrane of anterior nasal cavity), infraorbital nerve (external nares), and sphenopalatine nerve (sensation to posterior and central nasal cavity).

The structural support of the internal and external nasal lining is conferred by a combination of bony and cartilaginous structures. The floor of the nose is made up of premaxilla and palatine bones. The paired nasal bones attach to the frontal bone superiorly at the rhinion, to the lacrimal bones superolaterally, and to the ascending process of the maxilla inferolaterally. The bony nasal septum, located posteriosuperiorly, is comprised of the perpendicular plate of the ethmoid bone; the vomer arises posteroinferiorly within the nose at the choana. The cartilaginous septum forms a quadrangular shape at the anterior septum. The upper lateral cartilages lie lateral to the septum and fuse at the dorsal septum; they are adherent to the pyriform aperture by loose ligamentous connections, while the inferior ends are not bound to another structure. The lower lateral cartilages are caudad to the upper laterals and they are complex paired structures with medial crura, which are associated with the caudal septum, and lateral crura that flair out from the caudal septum as support for lateral portion of the nostril.[18]

In addition to the cosmetic role that the nose plays, several functional points must be emphasized. In a basic sense, the nose acts to humidify, filter, and warm air as it is inhaled. The mucosa with its mucous secreting glands and the ciliated epithelium are adept at removing particulate matter from inhaled air and passing it posteriorly where it can be expectorated or swallowed in mucous. The lateral nasal wall structure contains the sinus ostia, which depend on normally functioning epithelium for drainage. The narrowest segment of nasal airway is the nasal valve where the nasal septum meets the upper lateral cartilage at the dorsum of the nose. In total nasal reconstruction, the goals should be to maintain sinus drainage when possible, preserve functional mucosa where it remains, and reconstitute an adequate nasal airway.

ETIOLOGY OF THE MODERN TOTAL NASAL DEFECT

Five broad categories are inclusive of most known causes of nasal defects: traumatic, infectious, toxic, inflammatory, and neoplastic. Most conditions that fall within these categories will not go on to create a total nasal defect, however, a working knowledge of causative conditions is essential to identify those patients in need of further care for infectious diseases, inflammatory conditions, substance abuse, psychiatric illness, or cancer (**Table 1**).[20]

The most common causes of the total nasal defect today are trauma or cancer resections.[21] In both cases, unique sets of wound healing and cancer surveillance issues arise that may serve to delay reconstruction. After trauma, especially after blast-wounds such as gunshots to the face during civilian or military conflict, it is critical to debride the wound and allow tissue in process of necrosis to declare itself while stabilizing remaining structures and soft tissues of the face in the initial encounter. Subsequent encounters are focused upon reconstruction of the damaged structures and refinement to optimize function and aesthetics.[22] Alternatively, massive soft tissue defects can result from skin cancer resections and may result in total nasal defect. Immediate reconstruction of cancer defects was initially controversial with several authors arguing for one to two year delays in reconstruction secondary to relatively high rates of recurrence (30%).[13,14] However, more recently, the advent of Mohs microsurgical resection has afforded a lower recurrence rate for nonmelanoma skin cancer even with three-dimensional resections such as with the nose; this success weakens the argument for delaying reconstruction when the social morbidity of delaying is high.[23] Therefore, most ablative/reconstructive teams now perform the initial reconstruction at the same time as the resection—even in the case of massive skin tumors that require microvascular tissue transfers.[24]

RECONSTRUCTION OF THE TOTAL NASAL DEFECT

The decision to perform reconstruction or prosthesis rests with the patient at the counsel of the consulting physician. Depending on the patients' overall health and desire to avoid a prosthetic, they may or may not be motivated to undergo further procedures involved with reconstructing the nose. The prosthesis provides a reasonable alternative to surgical repair, and this option should be afforded the patient before they consent to a procedure. If the patient desires surgical alternatives, a total nasal defect reconstruction should include reconstituting each of the three layers of nasal tissue (ie, the inner lining skin and mucosa, and the structural support of bone and cartilage) to give the lining lasting form and an external envelope of skin. The surgical approaches and techniques for each layer are explored below.

Table 1
Etiology of modern destructive nasal processes

Category	Diagnoses	
Traumatic	Animal or human bite Accident Iatrogenic (surgical) Self-induced (rhiotillexomania)	—
Infectious	Bacterial:	Mycobacteria Syphilis Rhinoscleroma Leprosy Actinomycoses
	Fungal	Aspergillosis Rhinomucomycosis
Toxic	Cocaine abuse Chromium salts	—
Inflammatory	Sarcoidosis Foreign-body granuloma Wegener's granulomatosis Poly artritits nodosa Systemic lupus Hypersensitivity angiitis	—
Neoplastic	Skin cancers	Basal cell carcinoma Squamous cell carcinoma
	Sinonasal tumors:	Ethesioneuroblastoma Sqamous cell carcinoma
	Orbital tumors:	Rabdomyosarcoma
	Lymphoma:	Sinonasal non-Hodgkin's T-cell lymphoma

Data from Borges A, Fink J, Villablanca P, et al. Midline destructive lesions of the sinonasal tract: simplified terminology based on histopathologic criteria. AJNR Am J Neuroradiolo 2000:21:331–6.

Inner Lining

The natural inner nasal lining serves the important function of mucociliary transport, moistening, and humidifying the inhaled air. In addition, proper relative tissue volume is critical to allow for a nasal airway to be reformed. Multiple strategies have been devised for reconstruction of the total nasal defect; these strategies evolved from the experience of reconstructing partial and near-total defects (**Table 2**).[6]

Options include: skin grafts, mucosal flaps, local skin flaps, and free flaps.[5,6,8,11,17,24–30] Full or split-thickness skin grafts have been used to reconstruct the inner lining. Both types are thin but transfer epithelium into a natively moist place that results in troublesome dryness and crusting within the new nose. A variety of nasal saline irrigations are available to combat dryness, however, as Burget and Menick have argued in the past, like tissue is optimal for lining the nose.[8] One application of grafting that can be useful in settings where operative time requires limitation involves coupling a graft to a rotational or free flap in a staged fashion. The flap can be elevated and a split thickness skin graft (STSG) placed on the undersurface of the pedicle or muscle and staged to allow inosculation and graft survival. This method requires the surgeon to stage the structural grafting until such time as the inner lining has become vascularized.[11,25,28]

Mucosal flaps may be based within the nose or within the oral cavity. The major advantage of mucosa is that it replaces mucosal nasal lining with like tissues, which maintain the moisture of the nose better than skin grafts. Among the nasal graft options, the mucoperichondrial flap can provide a fairly large vascularized mucous membrane axial pattern flap for transposition to the middle nasal vault and alar rim (**Fig. 2**).[8] If bilateral flaps are harvested, one must take care to leave vascularized mucosa over an adequate dorsal septal strut to prevent nasal collapse. Despite their obvious convenience, septal flaps: may not provide adequate tissue in the total nasal defect; are thin and fragile thus more easy to devascularize; and are difficult to harvest. Additional mucosal flaps have emerged in the past several

Table 2
Internal nasal lining reconstructive options: pros and cons

Flap or Graft	Type	Pros	Cons
Local flaps	Nasal turn-in	Local availability	Poor vascularity, thick; requires thinning
	Nasolabial	Local availability	Thick, multi-staged
	Paramedian forehead	Local availability/reliability	Thick, multi-staged
Grafts	FTSG	Ability to sculpt tissue	Needs vascular bed; requires staging of support
	STSG	Ability to sculpt tissue	Needs vascular bed; requires staging of support
	Chondrocutaneous	Ability to sculpt tissue	Limited size; needs vascular bed; unpredictable take
	Chondromucosal	Ability to sculpt tissue	Limited size; needs vascular bed; unpredictable take
Mucosal flaps	Bipedicle vestibular	Local availability	Small, not enough tissue for total nasal defects
	Bipedicle mucosal	Local availability	Small, not enough tissue for total nasal defects
	Septal mucoperichondrial	Local availability, versatile, cartilage	Bilateral usa results in septal perforation/cartilage loss
	FAMM	Axial, robust	Thick, may need thining
Free flaps	Prelaminated	Ability to sculpt tissue	Muti-staged, contracture may occur and distort
	Auricular helical	Good color texture match	Technically challenging, small vessels
	Dorsal metacarpal artery	Thin skin, shape mimics nose	Technically challenging, small vessels
	Radial forearm	Ample tissue, can be thinned later	Bulky at first, crusting/dry nose

Abbreviations: FTSG, full thickness skin graft; STSG, split thickness skin graft; FAMM, facial artery musculomucosal.
Data from Taghinia AH, Pribaz JJ. Complex nasal reconstruction. Plast Reconstr Surg 2008:121:15e–27e.

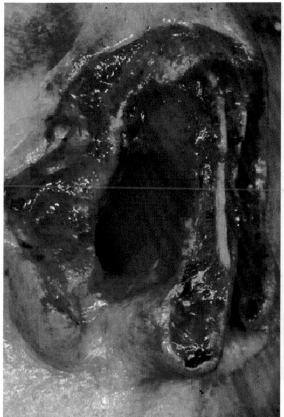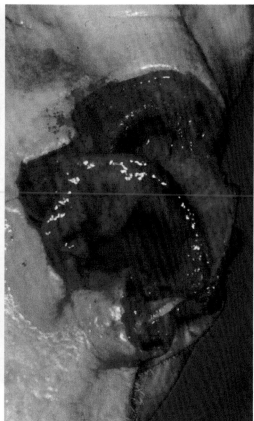

Fig. 2. Mucoperichondrial septal flap.

decades and serve as workhorses in local nasal reconstruction; among these, the inferior turbinate flap can provide comparable volumes of tissue to the septal flap.[31] In addition, some nasal processes such as cocaine use or vasculitic causes of nasal defects provide mucosa with compromised vascularity and thus alternative tissue is required.

One such option comes from the mucosa of the mouth: the facial artery muculomucosal flap (FAMM). It is an axial pattern flap first described by Pribaz and colleagues[32,33] based on the facial artery that can be transposed to the nasal cavity to provide mucosal lining that is both moist and well vascularized. It has even been shown useful in reconstruction of the Wegener's nose where vascularized nasal mucosa is at a premium.[34] The major disadvantage of the FAMM flap is bulk, which often will require subsequent thinning for nasal lining. In addition, the FAMM flap may not provide enough nasal lining to fill the total nasal defect even when harvested bilaterally, and thus may be used in combination with other local flaps. One must consider the vascular supply to the FAMM flap and ensure it does not interrupt critical

blood supply to other local flaps during planning of the reconstruction.

Lastly, a variety of regional turn-in, rotational, and transposition flaps have been described in reconstruction of the nasal lining (**Fig. 3**). The para-median forehead flap, melolabial flap, and random turn-in flap all transfer epithelial lining into the nose but are locally available.[35] The major disadvantages these flaps are the limited availability of tissue and transfer of dry skin, however, they may be used in concert with other techniques. Given the principle role of the forehead flap in reconstructing the envelope, most surgeons reserve its use for this layer.

One option for the total nasal defect that has been recently explored is the microvasular free flap. Authors began to explore free tissue transfer for this defect out of a desire to provide adequate volume of vascularized tissue for single stage reconstructions of the total nasal defect. In addition, it was recognized that when adjacent tissue of the face is resected, the free flap allows for additional tissue transfer and flexibility in reconstruction. In 2003, Winslow and colleagues described the use of free radial forearm facial flaps

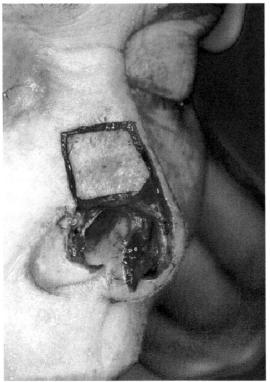

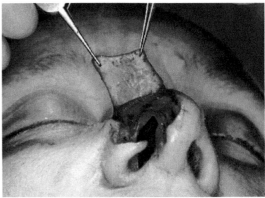

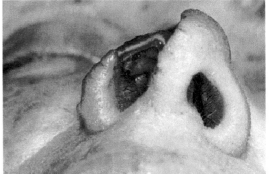

Fig. 3. Cutaneous turn-in flap.

to eliminate the transfer of intranasal epithelial tissue usually transferred with turn-in, regional skin flaps, or fasciocutaneous radial forearm flaps (**Fig. 4**). In addition, the authors have transferred osteocutaneous forearm flaps to assist with the structural layer of reconstruction.[5,26,27,30] Additional free flaps have been described for nasal lining and include the dorsal metacarpal artery flap[29] and the postauricular skin, with or without helical root cartilage and skin, based on the superficial temporal vessels.[36,37] However, the later two free flaps are more suited for external envelope reconstruction. Free flaps offer the advantage of bringing new vascularized tissue into the nasal vault to aid in the take of cartilage and bone grafts, resistance to planned post-operative radiotherapy, and the ability to graft free mucosa onto the vascularized free tissue with success. They are of particular advantage in cases where total defects are present that require replacement of large sections of nasal lining.[5]

Structural Support

After the inner lining has been reconstituted, the focus of reconstruction turns to the skeletal support. Without structural support, the reconstructed lining and envelope will not be aesthetic or functional. At a minimum, the reconstructed structure of the nose should resemble the preoperative nose. This result is accomplished by providing central structure to allow for tip projection and prevent midvault collapse and by contouring of the lateral subunits and alae to recreate distinct nasal features. Although graft material is available from the calvarium, septal cartilage and bone, rib, and auricular cartilage, the best combination of choices is case dependent. The technique used by the authors is described below, although alternative successful techniques have been described, which use other materials.[9]

Split calvarial bone and auricular cartilage are harvested in necessary quantities to provide adequate projection (similar to preoperative) and to provide enough cartilage to contour the nose. The calvarial bone is fashioned into an L-strut to the remaining nasal bones superiorly and the floor of the nose inferiorly and affixed with miniplates, thus creating central stability and the basis of a structural tripod. The auricular cartilage is then used to reconstitute the lateral sidewalls of the nose—with conchal bowl curvature used to the advantage of the surgeon—completing the tripod. A portion of helical root or conchal bowl may be

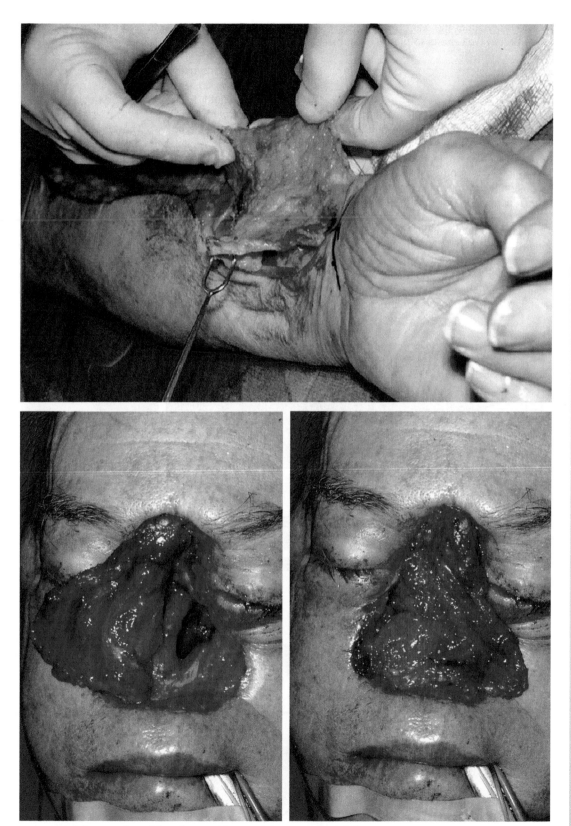

Fig. 4. Radial forearm fascial flap for nasal lining in the total nasal defect.

used to reconstruct the alar curvature, as well as create batten type grafts to prevent stenosis and contracture (**Fig. 5**).[5]

External Envelope

The last layer in of the reconstruction is the cutaneous covering to the support grafts and internal lining, ie, the envelope or external skin. Again, multiple options exist, including full and split thickness skin grafts, both of which lack good color match and which may distort shape with contracture. Transposition flaps that reconstruct part, but not all, of the total nasal defect tend to cross subunits and leave unsightly, noticeable scarring; options include melolabial flaps and cheek advancement flaps. Thus, the paramedian forehead flap, the oldest and most well described nasal reconstructive technique, remains the best local flap for total nasal reconstruction as well as for some partial defects and it will be the focus below.[7,38]

The forehead flap has the advantages of being an axial pattern flap with good color match to the nasal skin (**Fig. 6**). It can be created with ample length to reconstruct defects down to the columella or even parts of the internal nasal lining via infolding.[9,11] The flap is harvested based on the supratrochlear artery and vein; considerable variability in flap shape is possible, which makes it ideal for reconstruction of nasal defects of different sizes. In addition, the donor size can be largely closed primarily and heals favorably by secondary intention. The flap is harvested by first designing its shape using a template much the same as Suchrutu described in 400 BC. Some clinicians prefer to inject vasoconstrictors, although others feel it is disadvantageous to constrict circulation in the flap during harvest.

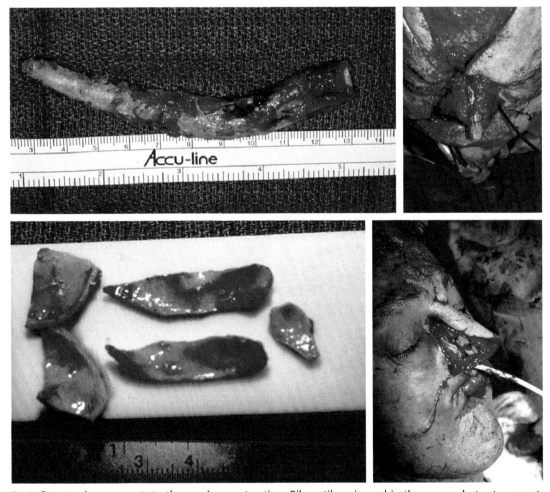

Fig. 5. Structural components to the nasal reconstruction. Rib cartilage is used in the upper photos to recreate central tripod. Lower photos show auricular cartilage use for lateral limbs of tripod and sculpting.

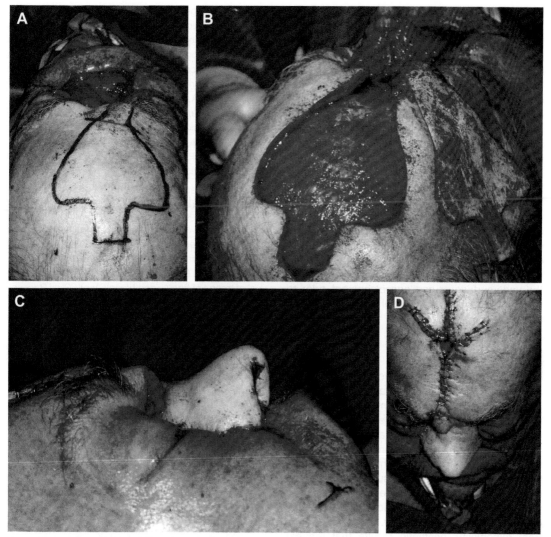

Fig. 6. Paramedian forehead flap design (*A*), elevation (*B*), inset and closure (*C*), and postoperative appearance (*D*).

First, an incision is made through skin, subcutaneous tissue, frontalis muscle, and galea until the periostium is encountered. Variations of the depth of harvest have been described with some surgeons preferring to harvest initially in a supragaleal plane until nearer to the pedicle. Next, the flap is elevated in a supraperiostial plan down to the level of the brow when more care must be taken to avoid injury to the pedicle. The pedicle is then identified and further dissection proximally can extend to below the brow for further rotation. The flap is then transposed into the defect by rotating it 180 degrees into the wound, while rotating it 90 degrees. Skin edges are approximated carefully and the donor site closed. The exposed pedicle can be maintained with moist gauze or xeroform, as can any open areas of forehead until pedicle division in 3 weeks. A disadvantage of the forehead flap is that it requires at least two, and usually three stages for refinement of the envelope.

At the second stage the pedicle is transected, and redundant tissue is either re-inserted into the donor site or discarded. The donor site is then closed primarily with care taken to maintain symmetry with the contralateral brow height. At the same setting, the proximal portion of the flap may be thinned, but dissection further than one-half the length of the flap may put its vascular supply at risk and is therefore not advised. The third setting involves further refinement of the re-constructed nose in the form of thinning in areas of bulk, recreation of an alar crease, and attempts to recreate subtle nasal features at the nasal tip. At this stage, it is also feasible to revise the nasal lining to provide a more adequate nasal airway if bulk is occluding the airway.

Special considerations include the use of bilateral forehead flaps to reconstruct the lining and envelope simultaneously. Or, in staged fashion, the forehead flap can be skin grafted on its undersurface over the frontalis muscle, then transposed with internal lining and envelope in a second stage.

Finally, free flap reconstruction of the envelope has also been employed. Some argue that the skin match with free tissue transfer is less ideal than a forehead flap, however, free flaps remain a viable option in some situations. Among the donor sites described are skin/ear free flaps based on the superficial temporal vessels, radial forearm (which can be prelaminated with skin grafting to the undersurface or cartilage placement prior to transfer to the face), and dorsal metacarpal artery flaps.[5,21,29,30,37]

SUMMARY

Total nasal construction has evolved considerably in the last 15 years to encompass more elegance and finesse. Whereas many defects were managed with a prosthetic nose, it is now feasible to provide patients with three-layered reconstruction that closely mimics the form and function of their natural nose. Through combined techniques that transfer local and free tissue to the face and nose it is now possible to line the nasal cavity, provide structural support, and add an external envelope safely and efficiently. Applying lessons from rhinoplasty, aesthetic results that respect anatomic borders and nasal subunits recreate a realistic appearing nasal reconstruction externally. Calvarial bone, septal, and auricular cartilage create the support and contour of the new nose. Local rotational flaps or free tissue can reline the nose. Ultimately, proper patient selection and a willing patient will allow for refinement over the course of multiple revision surgeries to ensure reconstitution of the nasal airway and aesthetic nose.

REFERENCES

1. Whitaker IS, Karoo RO, Spyrou G, et al. The birth of plastic surgery: the story of nasal reconstruction from the Edwin Smith Papyrus to the twenty-first century. Plast Reconstr Surg 2007;120:327–36.
2. Yalamanchili H, Sclafani AP, Schaefer SD, et al. The path of nasal reconstruction: from ancient India to the present. Facial Plast Surg 2008;24:3–10.
3. Moolenburgh SE, Mureau MA, Duivenvoorden HJ, et al. Validation of a questionnaire assessing patient's aesthetic and functional outcome after nasal reconstruction: the patient NAFEQ-score. J Plast Reconstr Aesthet Surg 2008 Feb 8. [Epub ahead of print].
4. Mureau MA, Moolenburgh SE, Levendag PC, et al. Aesthetic and functional outcome following nasal reconstruction. Plast Reconstr Surg 2007;120:1217–27 [discussion: 28–30].
5. Winslow CP, Cook TA, Burke A, et al. Total nasal reconstruction: utility of the free radial forearm fascial flap. Arch Facial Plast Surg 2003;5:159–63.
6. Taghinia AH, Pribaz JJ. Complex nasal reconstruction. Plast Reconstr Surg 2008;121:15e–27e.
7. Menick FJ. Aesthetic refinements in use of forehead for nasal reconstruction: the paramedian forehead flap. Clin Plast Surg 1990;17:607–22.
8. Burget GC, Menick FJ. Nasal support and lining: the marriage of beauty and blood supply. Plast Reconstr Surg 1989;84:189–202.
9. Burget GC, Walton RL. Optimal use of microvascular free flaps, cartilage grafts, and a paramedian forehead flap for aesthetic reconstruction of the nose and adjacent facial units. Plast Reconstr Surg 2007;120:1171–207 [discussion: 208–16].
10. Menick FJ. A 10-year experience in nasal reconstruction with the three-stage forehead flap. Plast Reconstr Surg 2002;109:1839–55 [discussion: 56–61].
11. Menick FJ. A new modified method for nasal lining: the Menick technique for folded lining. J Surg Oncol 2006;94:509–14.
12. Millard DR Jr. Total reconstructive rhinoplasty and a missing link. Plast Reconstr Surg 1966;37:167–83.
13. Teichgraeber JF, Goepfert H. Rhinectomy: timing and reconstruction. Otolaryngol Head Neck Surg 1990;102:362–9.
14. Stanley RJ, Olsen KD. Rhinectomy for malignant disease. A 20-year experience. Arch Otolaryngol Head Neck Surg 1988;114:1307–11.
15. Burget GC, Menick FJ. The subunit principle in nasal reconstruction. Plast Reconstr Surg 1985;76:239–47.
16. Millard DR Jr. Aesthetic reconstructive rhinoplasty. Clin Plast Surg 1981;8:169–75.
17. Baker S. Major nasal reconstruction. In: Papel ID, editor. Facial plastic and reconstuctive surgery. New York: Thieme Medical Publishers, Inc.; 2002. p. 601–14.
18. Tardy ME. Surgical anatomy of the nose. New York: Lippincott-Raven; 1990. p. 1–98.
19. Bolger W. Anatomy of the paranasal sinuses. In: Kennedy DW, Zinreich J, Bolger WE, editors. Diseases of the sinuses: diagnosis and management. Hamilton (ON): BC Decker; 2000. p. 1–11.
20. Borges A, Fink J, Villablanca P, et al. Midline destructive lesions of the sinonasal tract: simplified

terminology based on histopathologic criteria. AJNR Am J Neuroradiol 2000;21:331–6.

21. Ross CTA, Wax MK. Total nasal reconstruction using microvascular and pedicle tissue transfer - a three year experience. Phoenix (AZ): Triological Society, COSM; 2004.

22. Futran ND, Farwell DG, Smith RB, et al. Definitive management of severe facial trauma utilizing free tissue transfer. Otolaryngol Head Neck Surg 2005; 132:75–85.

23. Lang PG Jr. The role of Mohs' micrographic surgery in the management of skin cancer and a perspective on the management of the surgical defect. Clin Plast Surg 2004;31:5–31.

24. Wax MK, Burkey BB, Bascom D, et al. The role of free tissue transfer in the reconstruction of massive neglected skin cancers of the head and neck. Arch Facial Plast Surg 2003;5:479–82.

25. Menick FJ. The use of skin grafts for nasal lining. Clin Plast Surg 2001;28:311–21, viii.

26. Moore EJ, Strome SA, Kasperbauer JL, et al. Vascularized radial forearm free tissue transfer for lining in nasal reconstruction. Laryngoscope 2003;113:2078–85.

27. Koshima I, Tsutsui T, Nanba Y, et al. Free radial forearm osteocutaneous perforator flap for reconstruction of total nasal defects. J Reconstr Microsurg 2002;18:585–8 [discussion: 89–90].

28. Sinha M, Scott JR, Watson SB. Prelaminated free radial forearm flap for a total nasal reconstruction. J Plast Reconstr Aesthet Surg 2008;61:953–7.

29. Beahm EK, Walton RL, Burget GC. Free first dorsal metacarpal artery flap for nasal lining. Microsurgery 2005;25:551–5.

30. Walton RL, Burget GC, Beahm EK. Microsurgical reconstruction of the nasal lining. Plast Reconstr Surg 2005;115:1813–29.

31. Murakami CS, Kriet JD, Ierokomos AP. Nasal reconstruction using the inferior turbinate mucosal flap. Arch Facial Plast Surg 1999;1:97–100.

32. Heller JB, Gabbay JS, Trussler A, et al. Repair of large nasal septal perforations using facial artery musculomucosal (FAMM) flap. Ann Plast Surg 2005;55:456–9.

33. Pribaz J, Stephens W, Crespo L, et al. A new intraoral flap: facial artery musculomucosal (FAMM) flap. Plast Reconstr Surg 1992;90:421–9.

34. Duffy FJ Jr, Rossi RM, Pribaz JJ. Reconstruction of Wegener's nasal deformity using bilateral facial artery musculomucosal flaps. Plast Reconstr Surg 1998;101:1330–3.

35. Park SS, Cook TA, Wang TD. The epithelial 'turn-in' flap in nasal reconstruction. Arch Otolaryngol Head Neck Surg 1995;121:1122–7.

36. Pribaz JJ, Falco N. Nasal reconstruction with auricular microvascular transplant. Ann Plast Surg 1993; 31:289–97.

37. Swartz WM. Microvascular approaches to nasal reconstruction. Microsurgery 1988;9:150–3.

38. Menick FJ. Nasal reconstruction: forehead flap. Plast Reconstr Surg 2004;113:100E–11E.

Microvascular Reconstruction of Major Lip Defects

Michael J. Odell, MD, FRCS(C)[a],*, Mark A. Varvares, MD, FACS[a,b]

KEYWORDS

- Microvascular surgery • Free flap
- Head and neck cancer • Head and neck reconstruction
- Lip cancer • Lip reconstruction

FREE TISSUE RECONSTRUCTION OF LIP DEFECTS

The lip is a critical structure in terms of function and appearance. It is a highly complex organization of sensate skin, subcutaneous tissues, sphincteric muscle fibers, salivary apparatus, and mucosa. Loss of part or all of the lip can have severe functional or cosmetic sequelae. Reconstructive efforts must consider not only form and function but also the cultural background of patients, as there are significant differences throughout the world in what is considered ideal in terms of function and aesthetics. Reconstructive surgeons must have at their disposal a wide array of methods to restore the lip to a premorbid state as much as possible.

Non–Free Tissue Transfer Methods of Lip Reconstruction

Wherever possible, it is advisable and preferable to use local tissue to reconstruct lip defects. These tissues, as a general rule, provide the closest match in terms of skin color, thickness, pilosebaceous content, and functioning muscle that is available. A complete discussion of all these techniques is outside of the scope of this article. **Box 1** lists many of the available techniques.

Goals of Lip Reconstruction

Oral competence
Restoration of oral competence is a primary consideration when reconstruction of extensive lip defects is undertaken. Failure to establish an oral stoma that can seal itself effectively can have far-reaching consequences. Failure to seal can lead to a patient's inability to successfully eat foods with liquid or semisolid consistency effectively, which can have deleterious consequences in terms of nutrition. In severe cases, alternative methods of hydration and nutrition must be sought in the form of a gastrostomy tube. This can be avoided in most cases with careful surgical planning. Use of residual orbicularis oris muscle fibers can assist in creating a dynamic sphincter function, even when an adynamic tissue is used for reconstruction. Alternatively, reinnervated muscle can be used to augment any residual muscle function.

Cosmesis
The mouth is the focal point of the lower face from an aesthetic standpoint. Major ablative or traumatic defects often have devastating cosmetic and psychologic effects on a patient. Reconstructive efforts must consider this and every attempt should be made to carefully restore the lower face not only from a functional standpoint but also a cosmetic one. Patients who feel facially deformed often withdraw from social interaction and become depressed and reclusive. Patients' cosmetic goals and expectations must be assessed carefully before a reconstructive plan is finalized.

Avoidance of microstomia
Failure to create an adequately sized oral stoma can lead to multiple undesirable outcomes. In

[a] Department of Otolaryngology-Head and Neck Surgery, Saint Louis University School of Medicine, St. Louis, MO, USA
[b] Saint Louis University Cancer Center, St. Louis, MO, USA
* Corresponding author.
E-mail address: Modell2@slu.edu (M.J. Odell).

Facial Plast Surg Clin N Am 17 (2009) 203–209
doi:10.1016/j.fsc.2009.01.006
1064-7406/09/$ – see front matter © 2009 Elsevier Inc. All rights reserved.

those patients who have functional dentition, dental care can become difficult, or impossible, leading to uncontrolled dental and periodontal disease that can be difficult to treat because of lack of access. For those patients who do not have teeth, dental rehabilitation becomes impossible, secondary to the inability to introduce dental appliances through an overly narrowed opening. Both groups often have to modify dietary intake as a result of this. Although local flap reconstruction often is preferable to free tissue transfer, the reconstructive surgeon must not hesitate to apply microvascular techniques to avoid overly narrowing a patient's mouth.

Fasciocutaneous Flaps

Radial forearm
The radial forearm free flap (RFFF) is the mainstay of head and neck reconstruction. Based on the radial artery and the venae comitans or the cephalic vein, the RFFF is easy to harvest and has excellent vessel caliber and pedicle length. In addition, it can be harvested with the lateral antebrachial cutaneous nerve, which can be approximated to an appropriate nerve in the defect site in an attempt to provide sensation to the reconstructed site.[1-5] This can be especially important in lip reconstruction, where the sensation of drooling is critical to the biofeedback that goes into the total rehabilitation of the competent oral stoma.

Adequate reconstitution of the lip, in particular the lower lip, is facilitated by inclusion of the palmaris longus (PL) tendon in the harvest of the RFFF. This tendon is present in more than 90% of patients. It originates from the lateral epicondyle of the humerus and inserts into the palmar aponeurosis. Its function is to flex the wrist, a function duplicated by the flexi carpi muscle group. Sacrifice of the palmaris results in little or no functional deficit. Once harvested, the PL tendon provides an excellent sling, holding appropriately placed sutures. It can be sutured to the remaining orbicularis muscle and the modiolus to support the reconstructed lower lip and provide some dynamic closure of the oral stoma during contraction of the residual orbicularis oris (**Figs. 1–7**).

Anterolateral thigh
The anterolateral thigh (ALT) free flap has assumed increasing importance in head and neck reconstruction in recent years. Combining a large amount of tissue that includes skin, fascia, muscle, and nerve with minimal donor-site morbidity and little or no potential for limb ischemia after harvest, the ALT offers many desirable traits for reconstructive surgeons. First described by Song in 1984,[6] many reports have subsequently surfaced

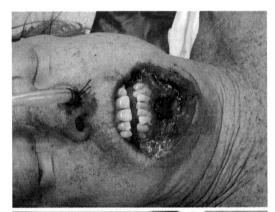

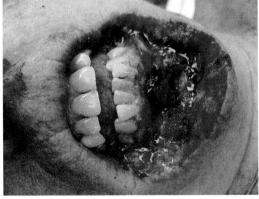

Fig. 1. Ablative defect in a 69-year-old woman after Mohs' micrographic removal of a recurrent squamous cell carcinoma of the lower lip and adjacent cheek.

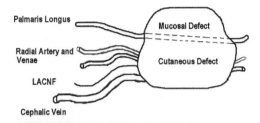

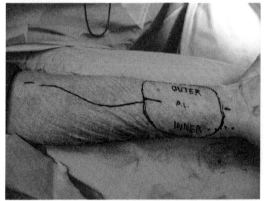

Fig. 2. Schematic of proposed use of the RFFF with PL tendon and RFFF donor site.

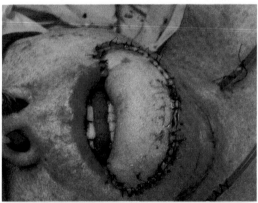

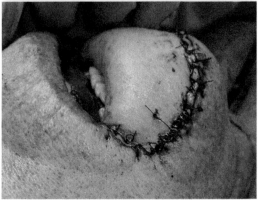

Fig. 3. Appearance at end of case.

regarding the use of this highly versatile flap.[7–11] The ALT shares many advantageous attributes with the RFFF, including thin, pliable tissue with the potential for cutaneous reinnervation. Most would agree that donor-site morbidity is better tolerated than the RFFF, as it consists of a simple linear scar. Split-thickness skin grafts rarely are necessary. The thickness of the ALT is dependent on body habitus. This is an important consideration for lip reconstruction, where thin tissue is preferable. As body mass index (BMI) increases, the ALT becomes less appealing for those sites that require thin tissue. The subcutaneous distribution also varies somewhat; women often have a slightly thicker ALT than age- and BMI-matched male counterparts.

The ALT is based on perforating vessels that originate from the descending branch of the lateral circumflex femoral artery and venae comitans. The exact configuration of the perforators can be variable,[12] leading to an occasionally technically challenging harvest. In addition, some perforators traverse a moderate amount of the vastus lateralis muscle before supplying the skin; meticulous (and sometimes tedious) dissection of these perforators from the surrounding muscle is necessary to minimize flap thickness. A single skin paddle can be fed by more than one perforator, which offers the opportunity to have multiple independent skin paddles.

With the presence of the thick fascia lata in the thigh, it is relatively straightforward to harvest vascularized or nonvascularized fascia for use as a sling, much in the same way that the PL tendon is used in conjunction with the RFFF.

Osteocutaneous Flaps

Composite defects of the lip and underlying bone pose unique challenges that often require increasing complex reconstructive efforts to achieve functional and aesthetic lip reconstruction.

Fibula

Since its introduction by Taylor in 1975,[13] the free fibula flap (FFF) increasingly has been used as the primary flap when vascularized bone is required as part of the reconstructive algorithm.

Based on the peroneal vessels, the FFF provides a large amount of strong bone with a good pedicle in terms of caliber and length. Its periosteal blood supply allows for multiple osteotomies, which confers unparalleled contouring ability. Harvest generally is straightforward and donor-site morbidity is acceptable to most patients. Preoperative evaluation must include documentation of good distal runoff from the

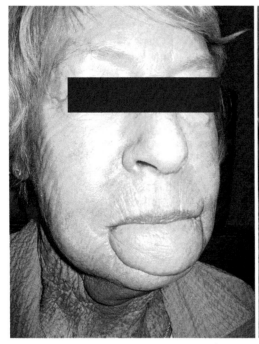
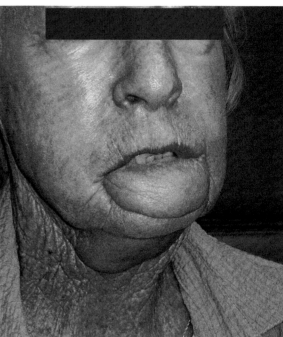

Fig. 4. Appearance 12 weeks postoperatively. Note that despite the patient's thin habitus, the flap would still benefit from debulking. She has achieved good oral competence and has a normal diet.

anterior and posterior tibial arteries to minimize the risk for foot ischemia after sacrifice of the peroneal. The FFF can be transferred as a sensate flap, using the lateral sural cutaneous nerve as the donor nerve. The fibular skin paddle can be divided in many cases or designed in a horizontal, rather than a vertical, configuration to better match a particular defect. All these factors make the FFF most surgeons' first choice for lip defects that also involve segmental mandibular or significant

maxillary loss. The fibula also can be used in conjunction with other soft tissue flaps for more complex defects.[14]

Osteocutaneous radial forearm

The radial forearm flap can be harvested with a segment of the radius to provide tissue for composite reconstruction. The benefits of the radial forearm flap are outlined in the first part of the section on fasciocutaneous flaps; it should

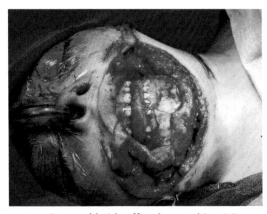

Fig. 5. A 3-year-old girl suffered an avulsion injury as a result of a dog bite. The injury was full thickness, down through the mandibular periosteum. It also involved approximately 30% of the upper lip, but the modiolus was partially intact bilaterally.

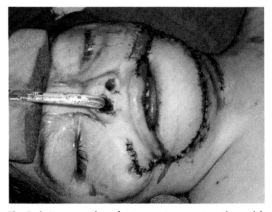

Fig. 6. Intraoperative photos post reconstruction with a RFFF and vascularized PL tendon. Note the left commissure has been reconstructed by advancing the buccal mucosa to cover the modiolus.

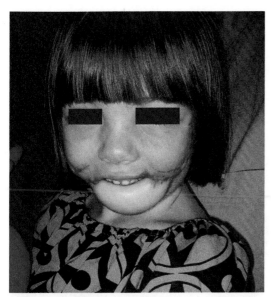

Fig. 7. Eight-week postoperative view. The lower lip has maintained height. The patient regained all weight lost after the injury on an oral diet and returned to preschool.

be reiterated that the thickness of this flap is, in general, ideally suited for lip reconstruction. Harvest of the osteocutaneous RFFF involves the inclusion of a pedicled section of distal radius with the overlying forearm skin. No more than 40% of the radius should be harvested to minimize the risk for excessive weakening of the major bony support of the wrist. Many surgeons apply a reconstruction plate in an effort to reinforce the remaining bone and further minimize the risk for pathologic fracture. The additional morbidity of bony harvest is minimal if care is taken during closure to avoid plate exposure.

The osteocutaneous radial forearm flap is ideally suited to the composite defect of the upper lip and premaxilla, where it is critical not only to restore the lip but also to provide bony support to avoid retraction of the upper lip into the premaxillary defect. Little bone is required. The radius easily can provide this without significantly increasing the risk for pathologic wrist fracture. Although the radius can provide a substantial amount of bone, many investigators prefer to use heavier bone stock for mandibular reconstruction.[15]

Subscapular system

The subscapular vascular system supports a variety of structures that have been used extensively in the reconstruction of myriad defects in the head and neck and elsewhere.[16] The unsurpassed versatility of the subscapular system allows for composite reconstruction of bony/soft

tissue defects with multiple bony, muscular, musculocutaneous, and fasciocutaneous paddles, all arising from the subscapular artery but with an independent blood supply. The primary uses of the subscapular system are the scapular fasciocutaneous or osteofasciocutaneous flap (based on the circumflex scapular artery) and the latissimus dorsi musculocutaneous flap (based on the thoracodorsal artery). Other components have been used in composite lip reconstruction, including the serratus anterior flap[17] and the scapular tip flap (**Fig. 8**). Although vessel caliber generally is excellent, more complex flap harvests generally result in a somewhat shorter vascular pedicle, which can necessitate the use of vein grafts, especially if the defect involves the midface and upper lip. Harvest difficulty varies, depending on the complexity of the flap. Patient habitus can be important; overweight or obese patients can have prohibitive amounts of subcutaneous adipose tissue, in the context of lip reconstruction. Donor-site issues are minor and generally involve subtle functional deficits of the upper extremity; these usually are greater when larger amounts of bone or muscle are harvested. Reliable sensate transfer of skin generally is not feasible for these flaps.

Dynamic Flaps

Gracilis

Restoration of a dynamic orbicular muscle sling always has been a primary consideration in lip reconstruction; this has led to attempts at using re-innervated muscle to restore a circumferential band of muscle after loss of the orbicularis oris. The most commonly cited[18–20] source of muscle is the gracilis. The gracilis muscle has been used extensively in the dynamic reconstruction of facial paralysis, congenital and acquired.[21,22]

The free gracilis flap is based on the adductor vessels, which themselves are branches of the profunda femoris; motor nerve input comes from the anterior branch of the obturator nerve. Harvest is relatively straightforward. Pedicle caliber and length are adequate but less than that of the RFFF. The gracilis does not have any substantial tendons in the area of the harvested muscle that are suitable for use as a sling.

The ability of this muscle to regain dynamic function after transfer is clear. The caliber of this muscle is well suited to lip reconstruction. Unfortunately, it cannot be transferred easily with a skin paddle for external or internal lining restoration; this has led to the use of local mucosal and skin grafting techniques to achieve reconstitution of all lip elements. Other efforts[18] have centered around the prefabrication of a mucosal lining before gracilis harvest

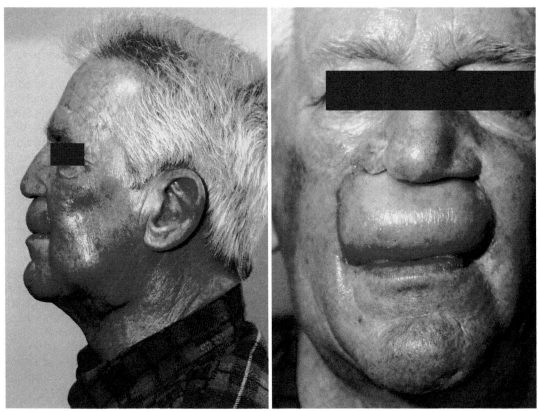

Fig. 8. Early postoperative view of RFFF used for upper lip reconstruction. The premaxilla was reconstructed using a tip of scapula/latissimus flap.

and transfer, obviating mucosal flaps. The effects of postoperative radiation on muscle reinervation after transfer are not clear.

SUMMARY

Reconstruction of extensive lip defects presents a significant challenge in terms of function and cosmesis; suboptimal results can have far-reaching consequences for patients. Having access to as many reconstructive tools as possible is critical to developing a comprehensive defect-based approach to lip restoration after major ablative or traumatic losses. The ultimate goal should be an adequately sized yet competent oral stoma that approximates the premorbid appearance as closely as is reasonable; this should allow patients to regain an acceptable quality of life after a potentially devastating illness or injury.

REFERENCES

1. Ozdemir R, Ortak T, Kocer U, et al. Total lower lip reconstruction using sensate composite radial forearm flap. J Craniofac Surg 2003;14(3):393–405.

2. Serletti JM, Tavin E, Moran SL, et al. Total lower lip reconstruction with a sensate composite radial forearm-palmaris longus free flap and a tongue flap. Plast Reconstr Surg 1997;99(2):559–61.

3. Jeng SF, Kuo YR, Wei FC, et al. Total lower lip reconstruction with a composite radial forearm-palmaris longus tendon flap: a clinical series. Plast Reconstr Surg 2004;113(1):19–23.

4. Carroll CM, Pathak I, Irish J, et al. Reconstruction of total lower lip and chin defects using the composite radial forearm–palmaris longus tendon free flap. Arch Facial Plast Surg 2000;2(1):53–6.

5. Cinar C, Arslan H, Ogur S. Reconstruction of massive lower lip defect with the composite radial forearm-palmaris longus free flap: empowered static and partial dynamic reconstruction. J Craniofac Surg 2007;18(1):237–41.

6. Song YG, Chen GZ, Song YL. The free thigh flap: a new free flap concept based on the septocutaneous artery. Br J Plast Surg 1984;37: 149–59.

7. Shieh SJ, Chiu HY, Yu JC, et al. Free anterolateral thigh flap for reconstruction of head and neck defects following cancer ablation. Plast Reconstr Surg 2000;105(7):2349–57.

8. Kimata Y, Uchiyama K, Ebihara S, et al. Versatility of the free anterolateral thigh flap for reconstruction of head and neck defects. Arch Otolaryngol Head Neck Surg 1997;123:1325–31.

9. Koshima I, Fukuda H, Yamamato H, et al. Free anterolateral thigh flaps for reconstruction of head and neck defects. Plast Reconstr Surg 1993;92:421–8.

10. Wei FC, Celik N, Chen HC, et al. Have we found an ideal soft tissue flap: an experience with 672 anterolateral thigh flaps. Plast Reconstr Surg 2002;109:2211–6.

11. Yildirim S, Gideroglu K, Aydogdu E, et al. Composite anterolateral thigh-fascia lata flap: a good alternative to radial forearm-palmaris longus flap for total lower lip reconstruction. Plast Reconstr Surg 2006;117(6): 2033–41.

12. Makitie AA, Beasley NJ, Neligan PC, et al. Head and neck reconstruction with anterolateral thigh flap. Otolaryngol Head Neck Surg 2003;129(5):547–55.

13. Taylor GI, Miller GD, Ham FJ. The free vascularized bone graft. A clinical extension of microvascular techniques. Plast Reconstr Surg 1975;55(5):533–44.

14. Kuzon WM Jr, Jejurikar S, Wilkins EG, et al. Double free-flap reconstruction of massive defects involving the lip, chin, and mandible. Microsurgery 1998; 18(6):372–8.

15. Militsakh ON, Werle A, Mohyuddin N, et al. Comparison of radial forearm with fibula and scapula osteocutaneous free flaps for oromandibular reconstruction. Arch Otolaryngol Head Neck Surg 2005;131(7):571–5.

16. Hallock GG. Permutations of combined free flaps using the subscapular system. J Reconstr Microsurg 1997;13(1):47–54.

17. Takushima A, Harii K, Asato H, et al. One-stage reconstruction of facial paralysis associated with skin/soft tissue defects using latissimus dorsi compound flap. J Plast Reconstr Aesthet Surg 2006;59(5):465–73.

18. Lengele BG, Testelin S, Bayet B, et al. Total lower lip functional reconstruction with a prefabricated gracilis muscle free flap. Int J Oral Maxillofac Surg 2004; 33(4):396–401.

19. Ninkovic M, di Spilimbergo SS, Ninkovic M. Lower lip reconstruction: introduction of a new procedure using a functioning gracilis muscle free flap. Plast Reconstr Surg 2007;119(5):1472–80.

20. Ueda K, Oba S, Ohtani K, et al. Functional lower lip reconstruction with a forearm flap combined with a free gracilis muscle transfer. J Plast Reconstr Aesthet Surg 2006;59(8): 867–70.

21. Zuker RM, Goldberg CS, Manktelow RT. Facial animation in children with Mobius syndrome after segmental gracilis muscle transplant. Plast Reconstr Surg 2000;106(1):1–8.

22. Zuker RM, Manktelow RT. Functional and aesthetic muscle transplants. In: Habal MB, editor, Advances in plastic and reconstructive surgery, vol. 9. St. Louis (MO): Mosby-Year Book; 1993. p. 37–66.

Reconstruction of the Midface and Maxilla

Mark G. Shrime, MD, FACS, Ralph W. Gilbert, MD, FRCSC*

KEYWORDS

- Maxilla • Reconstruction • Iliac crest
- Fibula • Scapula • Local flap

The functional and aesthetic importance of the maxilla is difficult to overestimate. The central face, nose, upper lip, orbit, malar region, and cheek form the centerpiece of facial identity. In addition, the maxilla mitigates transmission of occlusal forces to the cranium; supports the upper portion of the face, the cranial vault, and the brain; anchors the dentition; and forms the framework for the soft tissues of the face and muscles of facial expression. Loss of tissue volume or structural integrity in this region has far-reaching implications on mimesis, function, and aesthetic appearance.

Tumors affecting this region are disparate in pathology and behavior: squamous cell carcinomas arising from the epithelial lining of the palate, nasal cavity, and sinuses; primary orbital tumors; neoplasms of the minor salivary glands dispersed throughout the maxilla; midline destructive lesions; and mucosal melanomas make up the majority of the neoplasms affecting this region, in addition to benign odontogenic and nonodontogenic tumors and metastases from distant sites.[1–3] As a result, treatment varies, and the resultant defects from surgical resections span the spectrum from simple excisions to wide-field resections limited only by the dura above and the tongue below. Morbidity from these resections can be significant, not only affecting appearance and the structural integrity of the head but also engendering functional defects in swallowing, taste, speech, and vision.

Reconstruction of these defects, therefore, has been a matter of significant controversy. The goals of reconstruction must include the replacement of native tissue, the creation of a barrier between the oral cavity and structures superior to it, the reconstruction of maxillary architecture and the restoration of its structural integrity, the restitution of midfacial contour, the re-establishment of a scaffold against which the soft tissues of the face may be suspended, and, finally, the restoration of dentition and the return of normal masticatory function. Traditionally, maxillectomy defects have been reconstructed with prosthetic obturation. This reconstructive technique has many advantages, including the ability to restore contour, function, and a barrier between the oral cavity and the regions superior to it. For well over a century, obturation was the standard reconstruction for maxillary defects—Grover Cleveland, the 22nd and 24th President of the United States, famously was fitted with a rubber prosthesis after Dr. Joseph Bryant resected a malignant lesion on his hard palate in 1893.[4] Despite its advantages, however, obturation has its own drawbacks, including the need for manual dexterity to maintain the prosthetic, the difficulty of obtaining perfectly leak-tight separation of the oral cavity from the nasal cavity and sinuses, the problem—depending on the amount of tissue resected—with long-term retention, constant irritation, and, of greatest import, decreased patient satisfaction.[5]

In an attempt to mitigate these difficulties, reconstructive options have spanned the entire reconstructive ladder, with split- and full-thickness skin grafts, local flaps, pedicled regional flaps, and microvascular free tissue transfer all advocated. The choice of reconstruction depends most intimately on the size and location of the defect. The advent of microvascular reconstructive techniques has made the maxilla a region of significant innovation and advancement. Local

Wharton Head and Neck Centre, Princess Margaret Hospital, Toronto, Ontario, Canada
* Corresponding author.
E-mail address: ralph.gilbert@uhn.on.ca (R.W. Gilbert).

Facial Plast Surg Clin N Am 17 (2009) 211–223
doi:10.1016/j.fsc.2009.01.008
1064-7406/09/$ – see front matter © 2009 Published by Elsevier Inc.

facialplastic.theclinics.com

flaps can be used for small defects of the palate where the defect size would not allow prosthetic retention. Larger defects involving bone and those with loss of structural integrity are candidates for composite flap reconstruction.

CLASSIFICATION SYSTEMS OF MAXILLARY DEFECTS

Because of the complexity of the possible defects involved in the maxilla, multiple classification schemes have been proposed to aid in the choice of reconstructive options. Each scheme approaches the problem from a slightly different angle and no single scheme has achieved universal acceptance.

The earliest and simplest classification scheme for diseases of the maxilla was proposed by Öhngren in 1933. Because Öhngren did not believe that radical extirpation of maxillary tumors was effective therapy, favoring radiation treatment instead, his concern was prognostic and, as a result, his classification scheme placed little emphasis on maxillectomy defects. Instead, he famously split the maxilla in two, based on an imaginary line running from the angle of the mandible to the medial canthus of the ipsilateral eye;[6] tumors occurring anteroinferior to that line were believed to be "topographically more benign;" those posterosuperior to it were more lethal.[7]

The first classification to take surgical defects into account was proposed by Aramany in 1978.[8] Six different types of maxillectomy defects were identified:

1. The resection in the class I defect did not cross the midline and preserved the teeth on the contralateral side of the maxillary arch.
2. Class II defects were more limited, with preservation of the contralateral maxillary teeth, the central incisors, and, if possible, the canines and premolars on the resection side.
3. Class III defects involved only the central hard palate, without resection of any teeth.
4. Class IV defects crossed the midline, preserving only the posterior teeth on the contralateral side.
5. Class V defects involved resections of the posterior portion of the maxillary arch, with preservation of the mesial abutment teeth on both sides.
6. Finally, class VI defects involved resection of the midline central maxilla, with preservation of the teeth posterior to those used for abutment.

These defects are summarized in **Fig. 1.**

This classification remained the standard for nearly 2 decades, until Spiro and colleagues[7] published a revised schema, based on a retrospective review of 403 maxillectomies performed over a 9-year period. Unlike his predecessor's, Spiro's proposal broke defects down by the procedure performed rather than by resultant tissue loss. Three types of procedures were permitted in this scheme: limited maxillectomy, subtotal maxillectomy, and total maxillectomy (with or without orbital exenteration). Limited maxillectomy was subdivided further into medial, lateral, anterior, and inferior types.

Within the following 4 years, three other methods to classify maxillectomy defects were proposed. In 2000, Brown and colleagues[9] proposed the first classification scheme since Aramany's that focused on tissue loss. This scheme also proposed reconstructive techniques for each defect. In the Brown classification system, appraisal occurs of the vertical (classes 1–4) and horizontal (classes a–c) components of the tissue defect. Class 1 vertical defects cause no oroantral fistula; class 2 defects remain low; class 3 defects are high maxillectomies; and class 4 defects are radical maxillectomies with involvement of the orbit. Horizontal defects remain on one side of the midline without involving the nasal septum (class a), cross the midline or involve the nasal septum (class b), or involve resection of the entire hard palate and alveolar maxilla (class c). This classification scheme and the proposed reconstructive options are shown in **Fig. 2.**

In the same year, Cordeiro and Santamaria[10] expanded on the 1997 Spiro classification scheme, subdividing maxillectomies into partial/limited (type I), subtotal (type II), total with preservation of orbital contents (type IIIa), total with orbital exenteration (type IIIb), and orbitomaxillectomy (type IV). Type I maxillectomies involved resection of only one or two walls of the maxilla, not including the hard palate. Type II defects involved resection of five of the six walls of the maxilla (hard palate, anterior, posterior, lateral, and medial walls), with preservation of the floor of the orbit. Type IIIa defects involved resection of all six walls of the maxilla with preservation of the orbital contents; type IIIb involved sacrifice of those contents. Finally, type IV maxillectomies involved resection of the upper five walls of the maxilla (orbital floor, anterior, posterior, lateral, and medial walls) and the contents of the orbit, with preservation of the hard palate.

Based on experience with 60 patients in the span of 6 years, the investigators proposed various reconstructive options for these four types of maxillectomy defects. The classification

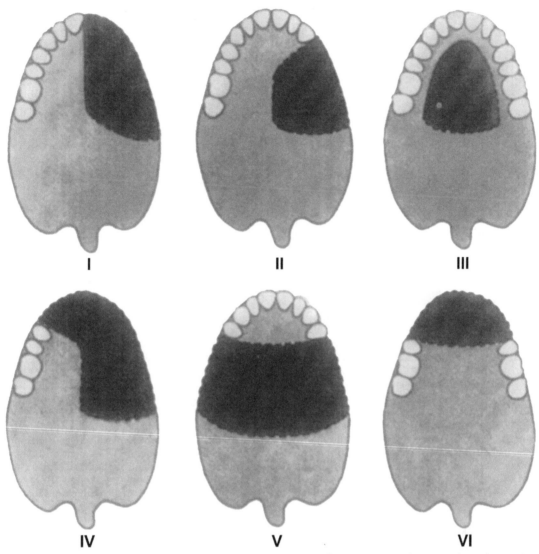

Fig. 1. The Aramany classification of maxillary defects. Class I: midline resection. Class II: unilateral resection. Class III: central resection. Class IV: bilateral anteroposterior resection. Class V: posterior resection. Class VI: anterior resection. (*Reprinted from* Aramany M. Basic principles of obturator design for partially edentulous patients. Part I: classification. J Prosthet Dent 1978;40(5):554–7; with permission.)

scheme and these reconstructive options are summarized in **Table 1**.

In 2001, Okay and colleagues[11] proposed a maxillectomy defect classification system with a view toward the assessment of functional outcome, prosthetic retention, and patient satisfaction. Based on a retrospective review of 47 consecutive maxillectomy defects, this classification scheme also was the first to take the status of the zygomatic arch and orbital floor into direct consideration. In the Okay classification, class Ia defects involve any portion of the hard palate except the tooth-bearing alveolus. Class Ib defects involve any portion of the maxilla with the

preservation of both canine teeth. Class II defects involve only one canine (except in the case of transverse anterior palatectomies that resect less than 50% of the hard palate). Class III defects involve the resection of both canines or greater than 50% of the hard palate. Subclasses f (orbital floor) and z (zygomatic arch) also involve resection of those particular structures. Specific to this classification scheme is a focus on reconstructive outcomes: class Ia and Ib defects, for example, can be reconstructed with soft tissue alone whereas class III defects cannot retain an obturator and require a reconstruction that allow dental rehabilitation. Because the Okay classification is

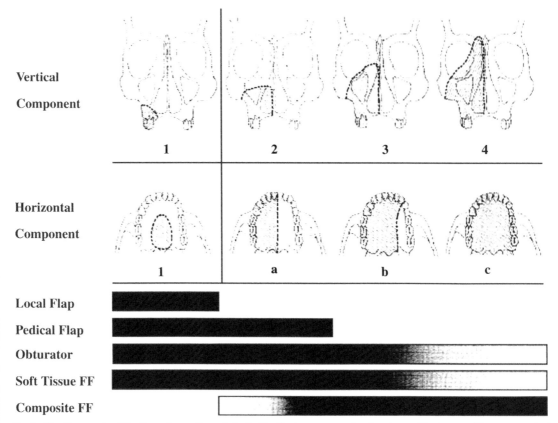

Fig. 2. The Brown classification of maxillary defects. Vertical component—class I: maxillectomy without oroantral fistula; class II: low maxillectomy; class III: high maxillectomy; and class IV: radical maxillectomy. Horizontal component—class a: less than or equal to half the hard palate and alveolus without involvement of the nasal septum; class b: greater than half of the hard palate and alveolus or involvement of the nasal septum; and class c: total hard palate and maxillary alveolus. FF, free flap. (*Reprinted from* Brown JS, Rogers SN, McNally DN, et al. A modified classifcation for the maxillectomy defect. Head Neck 2000;22:17–26; with permission.)

the only proposed scheme to focus on these outcomes, it is the one the authors favor. This classification is summarized in **Fig. 3**.

RECONSTRUCTIVE OPTIONS
Principles

As discussed previously, any reconstruction of the midface must, in addition to the restoration of form, restore as many of the functions of the native maxilla as possible. Speech, mastication, and swallowing must be re-established. Of prime importance to these functions, and especially to the former two, is dentition; any reconstructive option that prevents its restoration, therefore, should be avoided. For this reason, the reconstruction of an Okay class III defect with an obturator is counterproductive. Given the lack of abutment teeth in this defect, obturator retention is impossible, rendering the obturated patient an oral cripple. The same mode of thinking informs

decisions for the reconstruction of Okay class II defects. In jurisdictions in which dental implantation is feasible, these defects benefit from bony reconstructive options that allow such implantation; in the absence of this ability, these defects should be obturated. Finally, the reconstruction of large maxillectomy defects with soft tissue also is counterproductive in this regard: large soft tissue flaps quickly become ptotic, leading to denture mobility and poor long-term results.

Obturation

Obturation benefits from being customizable, sturdy, and safe from the effects of local tissue factors, which, in patients who have received radiation previously, can be significant. The reconstruction of a maxillectomy defect with an obturator, however, subjects patients to constant foreign-body irritation, the need for significant manual dexterity, a reconstruction that is never stable, and a lower quality of life. This latter factor

Table 1
Reconstructive procedures by maxillectomy type, Cordeiro classification

Type	Defect	Soft Tissue	Bone Source
I	Limited maxillectomy	Radial forearm Rectus abdominis Temporalis	Iliac crest
II	Subtotal maxillectomy	Radial forearm Rectus abdominis Radial forearm osseocutaneous Temporalis	Rib Vascularized radial graft
IIIa	Total maxillectomy	Rectus abdominis Temporalis	Rib Iliac crest Calvarium
IIIb	Total with orbital exenteration	Rectus abdominis	—
IV	Orbitomaxillectomy	Rectus abdominis	Rib

Data from Cordeiro PG, Santamaria E. A classification system and algorithm for reconstruction of maxillectomy and midface defects. Plast Reconstr Surg 2000;105:2331–46.

is significant: patient satisfaction with obturators for the closure of palatal defects is significantly lower than with a fasciocutaneous free flap reconstructive paradigm.[5] As a result, in patients who can tolerate longer operative times, other reconstructive options warrant consideration.

Local and Regional Flaps

Smaller defects, especially of the palate, present less of a cosmetic and structural deformity than do defects after formal maxillectomies. In these defects, return to normal function is of pre-eminent concern. Local flaps often are used, with minimal morbidity to the patient. Split- and full-thickness skin grafts have been used in the past[12] but their usage is limited by donor-site morbidity (especially with split-thickness grafts) and poor wound-healing properties at the recipient site, especially evident in graft contracture. As a result, their usage has become significantly less common. This section discusses the use of the palatal island flap, the buccal fat pad, and flaps based on the temporalis system. Other, less commonly used flaps, such as the submental island flap,[13] are not discussed.

Palatal island flap

In 1977, Gullane and Arena first described the palatal island flap for the reconstruction of small palatal defects.[14] This flap, based on the greater palatine vessels, may be used to resurface defects up to 15 cm^2 and is capable of restoring the oronasal barrier in through-and-through defects **(Fig. 4)**. It is limited by donor-site pain, but re-epithelialization of the donor site occurs within 3 months.[15]

Buccal fat pad

The buccal fat pad is a unique collection of adipocytes and stem cells within the buccal space, between the masseter and buccinators muscles, which has been used successfully for the reconstruction of smaller maxillectomy defects.[16,17] The vascular supply to this fat pad is surprisingly rich, allowing for rapid re-epithelialization and possibly for the use of this flap as lining in the setting of free, nonvascularized bone grafts.[18] The buccal fat pad is limited, however, by size; defects larger than 12 cm^2 are not amenable to this method of reconstruction.[17]

Temporalis muscle flap

When the resultant defect after a maxillectomy encompasses more than simply the palate, the structural functions of the maxilla and midface become paramount. Support of the cranium and, most especially, the remaining orbital contents, is required. Bony reconstructions are preferred; however, in patients in whom free tissue transfer is not a viable option, a rotational temporalis muscle flap, with or without nonvascularized bone, is a worthy surrogate. Because the natural curvature of the calvarium mimics that of the orbital floor, it can be used to reconstruct defects in the superior wall of the maxilla, with a rotational temporalis muscle flap for a vascularized bed. Access to the orbital floor, however, requires significant tunneling of the flap, putting the flap at risk for pressure-induced necrosis, or a partial

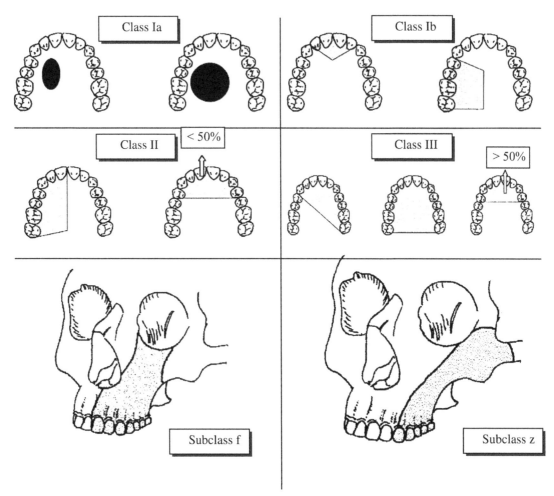

Fig. 3. The Okay classification of maxillary defects. Class Ia: no involvement of the tooth-bearing alveolus. Class Ib: preservation of both canines. Class II: resection of one canine or less than 50% of the hard palate. Class III: resection of both canines or greater than 50% of the hard palate. Subclass f: involvement of the orbital floor. Subclass z: involvement of the zygomatic arch. (*Reprinted from* Okay DJ, Genden E, Buchbinder D, et al. Prosthodontic guidelines for surgical reconstruction of the maxilla: a classification system of defects. J Prosthet Dent 2001;86:352–63; with permission.)

resection of the lateral portion of the zygomatic arch, risking weakening of the facial buttresses. In addition, because the frontal branch of the facial nerve crosses this arch, it also is placed at risk.

A temporoparietal osteofascial flap also has been described,[19,20] which provides the added benefits of allowing the transfer of vascularized bone to the orbital floor and affording a rotational flap with significantly less bulk than that harvested with the muscle flap, mitigating some of the difficulties discussed previously. The temporalis flap, however, suffers two significant disadvantages. For reconstructions of large palatal defects, in which the flap is asked to reach to the contralateral maxilla, there is a not insignificant rate of partial flap failure. In addition, the donor-site cosmetic

defect is significant and, unfortunately, relatively unavoidable. Despite its drawbacks, the temporalis system, when used appropriately, has proved a particularly effective and robust donor site for the reconstruction of maxillary defects,[21,22] with a low overall failure rate and a reproducible ability to withstand postoperative radiotherapy.

Free Tissue Transfer

With the advent of microvascular techniques and free tissue transfer, the reconstruction of the maxilla and midface has become an area of significant research and innovation.[23–25] The donor-site armamentarium available to microsurgeons for the reconstruction of the maxilla and midface is

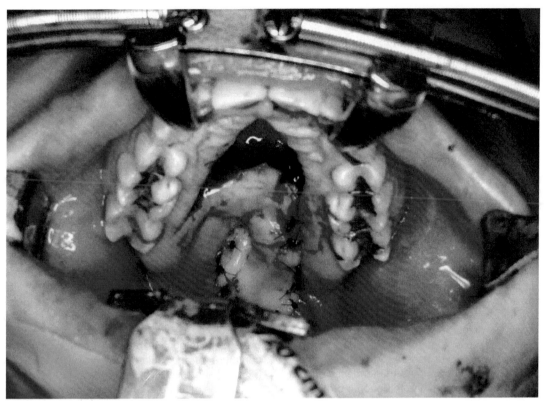

Fig. 4. A palatal reconstruction with the palatal island flap, based, in this patient, on the right greater palatine vascular pedicle. The anterior portion of this flap is left open to heal by secondary intention.

astonishingly diverse. Depending on the defect, fasciocutaneous, osteocutaneous, myocutaneous, myogenous, and myo-osseous flaps all are used in the reconstruction of maxillary defects.

The Radial Forearm System

There are many features of the radial forearm system that make it a good flap for head and neck reconstruction: its anatomy is relatively constant, its vascular pedicle long and of good caliber, and its harvest comparatively easy. It is primarily harvested, however, as a fasciocutaneous flap and, therefore, is suited most appropriately for smaller, less structurally significant defects. Its primary use as a fasciocutaneous flap has been for the reconstruction of Okay class Ia and Ib defects, in which the functional deficit engendered by the lack of separation of the oral and nasal cavities is the primary reconstructive concern. In that setting, as discussed previously, it offers equivalent patient satisfaction with taste, aesthetic appearance, and mastication as an obturator but affords patients improved satisfaction with social interaction, speech quality, comfort, and convenience.[5]

Despite the possibility of significant donor-site morbidity, including radial bone fracture,[26] the radial forearm system also has been harvested as an osseofasciocutaneous flap for the reconstruction of subtotal maxillectomy defects. In this setting, the radial forearm skin island is wrapped around the harvested portion of the radial bone, in a "sandwich" configuration. The osseous component is used for the reconstruction of the resected maxillary buttresses; the folded skin paddle reconstructs the oral and nasal lining.[10,26]

The Rectus Abdominis

What the rectus abdominis free flap lacks in vascularized bone, it makes up for in volume. A significant volume of muscle and adipose tissue can be harvested with this flap in addition to multiple, independent skin islands. Based on the deep inferior epigastric artery and its vein, and its cutaneous perforators, this flap also affords ease of harvest, constant anatomy, and a reliable vascular pedicle. Bone for the reconstruction of the orbital floor or maxillary buttresses, however, must be nonvascularized given the lack of available bone stock in the donor site. This prevents later

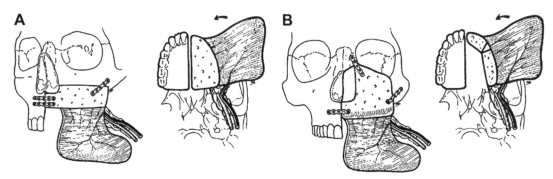

Fig. 5. (*A*) Reconstruction of a low maxillectomy defect using a horizontally oriented iliac crest free flap. (*B*) Reconstruction of a middle-height maxillectomy defect using a vertically oriented iliac crest free flap. Note that, in this case, the internal oblique muscle is rotated medially to close the resultant palatal defect. (*Reprinted from* Brown JS. Deep circumflex iliac artery free flap with internal oblique muscle as a new method of immediate reconstruction of maxillectomy defect. Head Neck 1996;18:412–21; with permission.)

osseointegrated dental implantation, but the flap has been successfully combined with the use of these nonvascularized bone grafts.[27] Although experience with this flap in the reconstruction of maxillary defects has been extensive, and aesthetic results tend to be favorable,[27,28] the authors do not favor its use, given its inability to offer structural support and the tendency of cutaneous portions of this flap to become ptotic.

The Fibula

The fibula has been used as a microvascular reconstructive option for the mandible and the maxilla; the bulk of experience in this flap has been with the former.[29] The fibula benefits from one of the greatest sources of bone stock available to the reconstructive microsurgeon: its bone is long, perfused by its nutrient arteries and a rich periosteal system—allowing for multiple osteotomies, and can accept osseointegrated dental implants. In addition, it can be accessed using a two-team approach and may be harvested as an osseous or an osseocutaneous flap. Its limitations, however, include a short vascular pedicle necessitating a vein graft in a large proportion of patients requiring the reconstruction of total maxillectomy defects, a not negligible donor-site functional morbidity, and the fact that modeling a straight long bone into the curved architecture of the maxilla is not always an easy undertaking.[24,25] In addition, modeling it to reconstruct the 3-D square frustum that is the maxilla is nearly impossible; thus, as the maxillectomy defect increases in complexity, the usefulness of the fibular free flap decreases.[30,31]

The Iliac Crest

The bone stock available from the iliac crest overcomes many of the limitations described

previously. Its bone is curved; it can be harvested with a significant muscular component if the internal oblique muscle is left attached; and it can be used to reconstruct low, middle, or high maxillectomy defects. For low defects, the iliac crest is oriented horizontally, reconstructing the curvature of the palate and maxillary alveolus (**Fig. 5**A). For middle defects involving the structures of the midface, the flap may be oriented vertically, reconstructing the maxillary buttress (**Fig. 5**B). In this situation, the internal oblique muscle is rotated internally and is itself used to close the palatal defect.[32] Re-epithelialization of this muscle is relatively rapid. Finally, for high

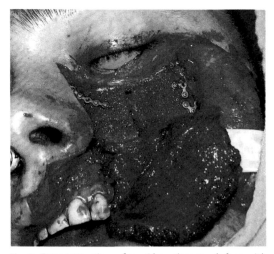

Fig. 6. Reconstruction of an Okay class II$_{fz}$ defect with a vertically oriented, split iliac crest graft. Nonvascularized bone was used to reconstruct the orbital floor and was plated to the vascularized portion of the graft. The internal oblique muscle is seen at the bottom of the picture; this was rotated posteriorly to reconstruct the palatal defect.

defects, the muscle itself may be used to obliterate the orbital defect. The bone stock available from the iliac crest also is sturdy enough to accept osseointegrated implants.[24,25,32]

Unfortunately, despite the benefits inherent to this flap, it has its limitations: the internal oblique muscle is comparatively tethered relative to the bone, and the length of the deep circumflex iliac artery and vein pedicle often is prohibitively short (approximately 4–5 cm), especially for higher defects. Although better than the long-bone options, the bone from the iliac crest is not ideally suited to the shape of the maxilla, and the flap often suffers from excess bulk. In addition, this donor site is fraught with significant morbidity, including pain, early difficulties with ambulation, and late risks for abdominal hernias.

A vertically oriented iliac crest reconstruction is shown in **Fig. 6**.

The Scapular System

Since its description in the mid-1980s as a potential microvascular donor site for head and neck reconstruction,[33,34] the scapular system has offered a plethora of reconstructive options. There are two osseous flaps that can be harvested off the vascular pedicle that this system offers. Classically, the lateral border of the scapula has been harvested based on a nutrient artery branch off the circumflex scapular system. This flap has the advantage of attached muscle with which it can be harvested, and a skin island, which is relatively mobile. The pedicle is short and the harvested

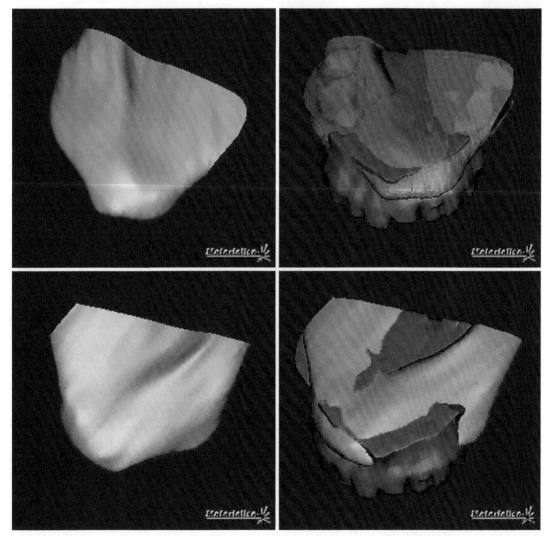

Fig. 7. CT conformance studies of scapular tip and palatal shape. The upper row shows conformance with the left scapular tip, the lower row with the right. In this patient, mean conformance distance was 2.04 mm (range 0.19–6.56 mm).

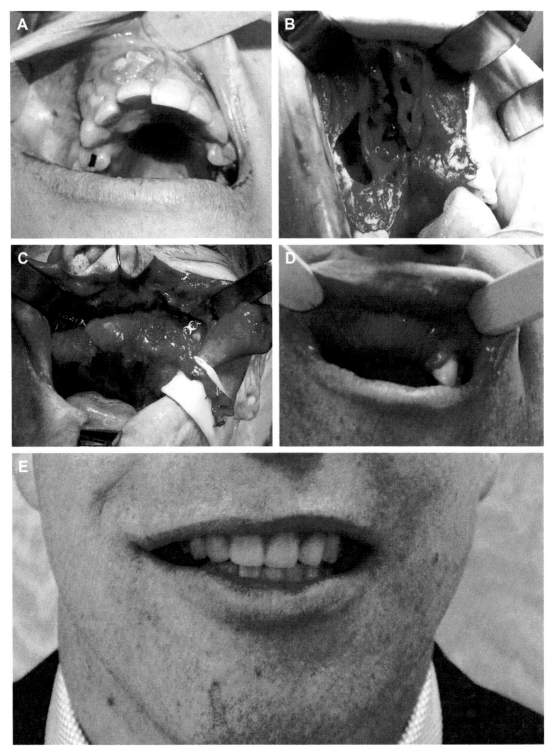

Fig. 8. Reconstruction of an Okay class II defect with a horizontally oriented scapular tip free flap. (*A*) The original osteosarcoma. (*B*) The defect after resection of the primary lesion. (*C*) Reconstruction with a horizontally oriented scapular tip; the angular artery pedicle is seen at the right of the image. (*D*) The reconstructed defect after mucosalization of the teres major muscle. (*E*) The fully rehabilitated result; this patient opted for denture reconstruction as opposed to dental implantation.

bone is rectangular, however. A second osseous flap was described by Coleman and Sultan in 1991.[35] Based on the angular artery, which branches off the serratus muscle branch of the thoracodorsal artery or off the main trunk itself with approximately equal frequency,[24] this flap centers on the scapular tip and offers multiple advantages over the standard scapular flap. The vascular pedicle is long (10–12 cm), a separate skin island can be harvested based on thoracodorsal artery perforators, the teres major muscle can be harvested along with the scapular tip, and the bone is ideally suited for reconstruction of vertical and horizontal maxillary defects (see discussion later). There is a rich collateral plexus between the angular artery and the circumflex scapular artery, and direct cutaneous branches off the thoracodorsal artery itself, allowing myriad reconstructive options.

More than any other flap discussed, the scapula is ideally suited for the reconstruction of the maxilla. The shape of the tip of the scapula conforms to the curvature of the maxilla nearly identically. In CT conformational studies, performed at the authors' institution, the average variance between the shape of the scapular tip and that of the palate is approximately 2.13 mm (range 0.21 to 8.51 mm), making the scapular tip a nearly perfect reconstructive modality for the maxilla (**Fig. 7**).

Similar to reconstruction using the iliac crest, the scapula can be positioned horizontally or vertically; the teres major muscle may be rotated medially to reconstruct palatal defects in the latter setting, in much the same way that the internal oblique is used in the iliac crest reconstructions. In addition, the midportion of the scapular body itself carries a curve similar to that of the orbital floor and, therefore, can be used as a nonvascularized graft for its reconstruction. Other benefits of this donor site over others (discussed previously) include minimal functional morbidity, an exceedingly long vascular pedicle, the ability to design multiple skin flaps based on the scapular and parascapular branches of the circumflex scapular artery and the thoracodorsal artery perforators, and a well-hidden scar. Limitations are few: the flap cannot be harvested in a two-team approach and often requires positioning that may make the initial ablative resection more difficult **Fig. 8**.

To date, the authors' institution has performed 29 reconstructions of maxillectomy defects with the angular artery/scapular tip free flap. (The first 14 of these have been reported in previous publications.)[36] Of these reconstructions, 24 were performed for malignant disease and five for benign disease. Fourteen patients had Okay class III defects, 10 class II, and 2 class I. Three patients had intact palates, with resections only of the orbital rim or zygomatic complex (a defect not classifiable using the Okay system). Mean hospital stay was 10.5 days, and three patients had significant medical complications (pulmonary embolus, respiratory failure, and death from an acute myocardial infarction). Four patients had donor-site seromas, and two required treatment for facial wound infections. No vein grafts were needed, speaking to the adequate length of the harvestable vascular pedicle. Six patients had a shallow vestibulobuccal sulcus, which was treated during a second procedure with a vestibuloplasty and split-thickness skin graft. Five patients suffered postoperative ectropion, and three had epiphora postoperatively; both complications were treated successfully in second procedures.

Eighteen patients agreed to undertake the Disabilities of the Arm, Shoulder and Head questionnaire.[37] On this questionnaire—a joint initiative of the American Academy of Orthopaedic Surgeons, the Council of Musculoskeletal Specialty Societies, and the Institute for Work & Health (in Toronto)—the normative score is 10.1. In the patients who completed the questionnaire, the mean score also was 10.1, supporting minimal donor-site functional morbidity from the harvest of the scapular tip.

Fourteen patients were able to return to a normal diet; 13 were able to wear dentures. Because of significant financial constraints surrounding the procedure, only two patients progressed to an attempt at osseointegrated implantation. One was implanted successfully and one was found to have inadequate bone stock.

The authors' experience has confirmed the significant usefulness gained from the use of free vascularized tissue from the scapular system in the reconstruction of maxillectomy defects. This system avoids many of the limitations inherent in other donor sites while maintaining or improving upon their advantages.

SUMMARY

The 3-D structure of the maxilla and its fundamental role in the structural and functional integrity of the face makes its reconstruction challenging and of primary import to a patient's aesthetic appearance, postoperative function, and overall satisfaction. There are myriad reconstructive options for maxillectomy defects, depending on the size and location of the defect. In keeping with the complexity of this area in the head and neck, no single classification encompasses all the possible defects concisely and perfectly reproducibly. Similarly, no single reconstructive option can be used for every defect. For larger defects, however, the bone-muscle flaps—namely, the iliac crest and the scapular tip—seem most ideally suited for this region of head and neck reconstruction.

REFERENCES

1. Kaneda T, Minami M, Kurabayashi T. Benign odontogenic tumors of the mandible and maxilla. Neuroimaging Clin N Am 2003;13:495–507.
2. Underhill TE, Katz JO, Pope TLJ, et al. Radiologic findings of diseases involving the maxilla and mandible. Am J Roentgenol 1992;159:345–50.
3. Weber AL, Bui C, Kaneda T. Malignant tumors of the mandible and maxilla. Neuroimaging Clin N Am 2003;13:509–24.
4. Keen W. The surgical operations on president Cleveland in 1893. Philadelphia: GW Jacobs & Co; 1917.
5. Genden E, Wallace DI, Okay DJ, et al. Reconstruction of the hard palate using the radial forearm free flap: indications and outcomes. Head Neck 2004;26:808–14.
6. Öhngren LG. Malignant tumors of the maxilloethmoidal region. Acta Otolaryngol 1933;19(Suppl):101–6.
7. Spiro RH, Strong EW, Shah JP. Maxillectomy and its classification. Head Neck 1997;19:309–14.
8. Aramany M. Basic principles of obturator design for partially edentulous patients. Part I: classification. J Prosthet Dent 1978;40(5):554–7.
9. Brown JS, Rogers SN, McNally DN, et al. A modified classifcation for the maxillectomy defect. Head Neck 2000;22:17–26.
10. Cordeiro PG, Santamaria E. A classification system and algorithm for reconstruction of maxillectomy and midface defects. Plast Reconstr Surg 2000;105:2331–46.
11. Okay DJ, Genden E, Buchbinder D, et al. Prosthodontic guidelines for surgical reconstruction of the maxilla: a classification system of defects. J Prosthet Dent 2001;86:352–63.
12. Rhee PH, Friedman CD, Ridge JA, et al. The use of processed allograft dermal matrix for intraoral resurfacing: an alternative to split thickness skin grafts. Arch Otolaryngol Head Neck Surg 1998;124:1201–4.
13. Genden E, Buchbinder D, Urken M. The submental island flap for palatal reconstruction: a novel technique. J Oral Maxillofac Surg 2004;62:387–90.
14. Gullane PJ, Arena S. Palatal island flap for reconstruction of oral defects. Arch Otolaryngol Head Neck Surg 1977;103:598–9.
15. Moore BA, Magdy E, Netterville JL, et al. Palatal reconstruction with the palatal island flap. Laryngoscope 2003;113:946–51.
16. Neder A. Use of buccal fat pad for grafts. Oral Surg Oral Med Oral Pathol 1983;55:349–50.
17. Arce K. Buccal fat pad in maxillary reconstruction. Atlas Oral Maxillofac Surg Clin North Am 2007;15:23–32.
18. Zhong LP, Chen GF, Fan LJ, et al. Immediate reconstruction of maxilla with bone grafts supported by pedicled buccal fat pad graft. Oral Surg Oral Med Oral Pathol 2004;97:147–54.
19. Choung PH, Nam IW, Kim KS. Vascularized bone grafts for mandibular and maxillary reconstruction: the pariental osteofascial flap. J Craniomaxillofac Surg 1991;19:235–42.
20. Parhiscar A, Har-El G, Turk JB, et al. Temporoparietal osteofascial flap for head and neck reconstruction. J Oral Maxillofac Surg 2002;60:619–22.
21. Abubaker AO, Abouzgia MB. The temporalis muscle flap in reconstruction of intraoral defects: an appraisal of the technique. Oral Surg Oral Med Oral Pathol 2002;94:24–30.
22. Ward B. Temporalis system in maxillary reconstruction: temporalis muscle and temporoparietal galea flaps. Atlas Oral Maxillofac Surg Clin North Am 2002;15:33–42.
23. Coskunfirat OK, Wei FC, Huang WC, et al. Microvascular free tissue transfer for treatment of osteoradionecrosis of the maxilla. Plast Reconstr Surg 2005;115:54–60.
24. Dalgorf D, Higgins K. Reconstruction of the midface and maxilla. Curr Opin Otolaryngol Head Neck Surg 2008;16:303–11.
25. Futran ND, Mendez E. Developments in reconstruction of midface and maxilla. Lancet Oncol 2006;7:249–58.
26. Andrades P, Rosenthal EL, Carroll WR, et al. Zygomaticomaxillary buttress reconstruction of midface defects with the osteocutaneous radial forearm free flap. Head Neck 2008;30:1295–302.
27. Bianchi B, Bertolini F, Ferrari S, et al. Maxillary reconstruction using the rectus abdominis free flap and bone grafts. Br J Oral Maxillofac Surg 2006;44:526–30.
28. Browne JD, Burke AJ. Benefits of routine maxillectomy and orbital reconstruction with the rectus abdominis free flap. Otolaryngol Head Neck Surg 1999;121:203–9.
29. Hidalgo D. Fibular free flap: a new method of mandible reconstruction. Plast Reconstr Surg 1989;84:71–9.
30. Futran ND, Wadsworth JT, Villaret D, et al. Midface reconstruction with the fibula free flap. Arch Otolaryngol Head Neck Surg 2002;128:161–6.
31. Kim DD, Dreher MA. The fibula free flap in maxillary reconstruction. Atlas Oral Maxillofac Surg Clin North Am 2007;15:13–22.
32. Brown JS. Deep circumflex iliac artery free flap with internal oblique muscle as a new method of immediate reconstruction of maxillectomy defect. Head Neck 1996;18:412–21.

33. dos Santos LF. The vascular anatomy and dissection of the free scapular flap. Plast Reconstr Surg 1984; 73:599–603.

34. Swartz WM, Banis JC, Newton ED, et al. The osteocutaneous scapular free flap for mandibular and maxillary reconstruction. Plast Reconstr Surg 1986; 77:530–45.

35. Coleman JJ, Sultan MR. The bipedicled osteocutaneous scapula flap: a new subscapular system flap. Plast Reconstr Surg 1991;87:682–92.

36. Clark JR, Vesely M, Gilbert RW. Scapular angle osteomyocutaneous flap in postmaxillectomy reconstruction: defect, reconstruction, shoulder function, and harvest technique. Head Neck 2008;30:10–20.

37. Hudak PL, Amadio PC, Bombardier C, The Upper Extremity Collaborative Group. Development of an upper extremity outcome measure: the DASH (Disabilities of the Arm, Shoulder, and Head). Am J Ind Med 1996;29:602–8.

Microvascular Reconstruction of the Orbital Complex

Jeffrey S. Moyer, MD, FACS[a], Douglas B. Chepeha, MD, FRCS(C)[a],
Mark E.P. Prince, MD, FRCS(C)[a], Theodoros N. Teknos, MD, FACS[b],*

KEYWORDS

• Free tissue transfer • Scapula • Radial forearm
• Closed cavity • Skull base • Orbital exenteration

Orbital exenteration includes removal of the globe and other orbital soft tissues and is frequently necessary when orbital and periorbital malignancies involve the orbit and curative surgery is planned. The most common cancer types resulting in orbital exenteration are squamous cell carcinoma, basal cell carcinoma, melanoma, and sebaceous cell carcinoma.[1–4] Early in the disease process, there may be no signs of orbital invasion, but as the disease process progresses, limitation of ocular motility and globe displacement frequently occur.

Large paranasal sinus tumors and neglected cutaneous malignancies often require, in addition to orbital exenteration, extensive resections that can include the mandible, maxilla, skull base, and dura. In addition to the obvious cosmetic issues involved in orbital exenteration and extensive craniofacial resections, life-threatening complications often occur if the reconstructive techniques are not durable and capable of withstanding adjuvant chemoradiation. The ability to separate the aerodigestive tract from intracranial contents is critical for the prevention of postoperative complications and typically requires a large volume of reliably vascularized tissue when repairing extensive resections.[5] In addition, bony defects that involve the orbital rim, malar eminence, or frontal bar should be repaired to prevent either orbital complications (if the eye is preserved) or significant cosmetic defects from the loss of normal facial architecture.[5] The reconstruction of maxillectomy defects that often accompany extensive orbito-sino-nasal malignancies must also address the palate to maintain proper deglutition and speech.

The ultimate decision on the method of reconstruction of the orbital complex is highly dependent on the extent and volume of the defect. Most large defects require free tissue transfer to meet effectively both the functional and cosmetic requirements of the reconstruction. Free tissue transfer has decreased the complication rate of extensive resections as compared with reconstructions performed with local or regional flaps. In addition, when local flaps are absent or of poor quality because of prior surgery or radiation, free tissue transfer may be the best reconstructive option for the recruitment of vascularized tissue and bone. Some defects are amenable to closure with local flaps, however, and granulation or skin grafting of the orbital cavity after exenteration can be a viable option in the properly selected patient. Local flaps, such as the pericranial flap, are also often used in conjunction with free tissue transfer to maximize the reconstruction.

The method of reconstruction should be tailored to the defect and the postoperative needs of the patient. An important decision in the approach to the orbital exenteration defect is whether or not to leave the cavity closed or open.[6] A closed cavity is defined as an approach that fills the orbital

[a] University of Michigan Medical Center, 1500 East Medical Center Drive, TC1904, Ann Arbor, MI 48109, USA
[b] The Ohio State University Medical Center, 456 West Tenth Avenue, Cramblett Hall, Suite 4A, Columbus, OH 43210, USA
* Corresponding author.
E-mail address: ted.teknos@osumc.edu (T.N. Teknos).

Facial Plast Surg Clin N Am 17 (2009) 225–237
doi:10.1016/j.fsc.2009.01.011

cavity with soft tissue to the level of the orbital rim to preserve volume and maintains or restores the three-dimensional bony architecture surrounding the defect. Closed cavity reconstructions also have the added advantage of using fat or muscle to reinforce the separation between intracranial and extracranial compartments when there is communication between the orbit and anterior cranial fossa. Open cavity reconstructions typically involve the use of granulation or skin grafts to line the exenteration cavity and are generally only indicated for defects that do not involve extensive resection of surrounding orbital bone or result in a communication with the anterior cranial fossa. A prosthesis can be used with an open cavity reconstruction, but these frequently are not used by the patient and an eye patch is often used instead.[3] This approach also offers better tumor surveillance of the surgical bed.

GOALS OF ORBITAL RECONSTRUCTION

The orbital complex is a multifaceted area comprised of both soft tissue and bone. The important bony architecture of the region is comprised of the supraorbital rim; infraorbital rim; lateral orbital wall (greater wing of the sphenoid); and malar eminence. Craniofacial resections or maxillectomy defects that include an orbital exenteration (or portions of the supporting structure of an intact globe) also frequently involve the horizontal and vertical buttresses of the upper third and middle third of the face and these regions must be addressed to maintain the integrity of the orbital complex. Maintenance of the relationships between the orbital suprastructure and the upper and middle thirds of the face are crucial for the correct alignment of facial relationships in both the horizontal and vertical dimensions. Recognizing the importance of these intricate relationships is central to understanding the goals for the reconstruction of the orbital complex.

The goals of orbital reconstruction are to (1) provide separation of the oral and nasal cavities and separation of the intracranial and extracranial spaces; (2) when the globe is preserved to maintain and restore orbital volume and function and prevent postoperative orbital complications; (3) maintain and restore the infraorbital rim, supraorbital rim and frontal bar, and malar contour; (4) maintain facial volume and symmetry and prevent distortion of surrounding tissues and anatomic landmarks; and (5) avoid ptosis and malposition of the repair.[6,7]

APPROACH TO ORBITAL RECONSTRUCTION

The approach to orbital and midface reconstruction has continued to evolve over the past 20 years

to achieve better reconstructive goals. Initial reconstructive attempts emphasized skin grafts and local flaps, such as pericranial, galeal, and galeopericranial flaps.[8–12] Pericranial flaps offer an excellent vascularized barrier between the anterior cranial fossa and the orbitosinonasal cavities and provide a suitable substrate for grafting. Large composite defects of the orbital complex frequently involve the anterior fossa, however, and important aesthetic and functional midfacial structures, such as the orbital rim, malar eminence, palate, and large areas of facial skin. Local flaps have limited usefulness for these larger defects because of limited volume, damage from previous treatments, and the lack of a large cutaneous component. Regional flaps, with their associated constraints from limited pedicle length, are infrequently useful for defects in this region. Alternatively, the use of free tissue transfer makes possible the movement of large volumes of vascularized tissue and bone that is both versatile and can withstand the impact of postsurgical radiation therapy.

Several strategies for the reconstruction of midfacial defects with free tissue transfer have emerged in the reconstructive literature. These approaches are typically based on the extent of the maxillectomy defect and address simultaneously the aesthetic and functional requirements of both the orbital and palatal defects. For total maxillectomy defects with the loss of the infraorbital rim and an intact globe, some authors advocate the use of a rectus abdominis myocutaneous free flap for coverage and obliteration of the maxillary cavity and reconstruction of the infraorbital rim with a nonvascularized bone graft.[13,14] Resorption of nonvascularized bone along the infraorbital rim can be problematic, however, with this approach. Alternatively, the scapula osseocutaneous free flap, with appropriate osteotomies, has been used for reconstruction of the infraorbital rim and palate in extensive midfacial defects.[15,16] Other authors have described the use of the iliac crest myo-osseous flap for the repair of total maxillectomy defects, but this approach can be limited by excessive bulk in certain patient populations and need for vein grafts because of a shortened pedicle.[17,18] Several publications have also described the use of the fibula osseocutaneous free flap to repair a variety of maxillary defects.[19–21]

The authors' general approach for complex orbital defects is to perform a closed orbital reconstruction, which generally offers an improved aesthetic result when compared with an open cavity with or without a prosthesis.[6,7] For patients with significant comorbidities who have defects that do not require separation between the intra-cranial and extracranial compartments and have local tissues of sufficient quality (ie, nonradiated), local flap reconstruction and skin grafting of the open cavity can be possible in selected cases. For these smaller defects of the orbital complex that do not involve a significant portion of the bony architecture (ie, infraorbital rim) or where maintenance of bony projection is not necessary, a closed approach with a radial forearm fasciocu-taneous flap is often preferable (particularly when an intracranial communication exists), because of the reliability of the reconstruction after adjuvant chemoradiation. For larger defects of the orbital complex that do not require vascularized bone, the latissimus dorsi myocutaneous flap, the rectus abdominis myocuteneous flap, or anterolateral fasciocutaneous flap (with or without significant portions of the vastus lateralis) can be used to ablate the defect. For defects of the orbital rim that are less than 30% to 40% of the entire rim, the authors typically use an osseocutaneous radial forearm flap to reconstruct the orbital complex. If the defect is in conjunction with a total maxillec-tomy defect, they restore the masticatory surface with a palatal prosthesis. Addressing the orbital and palatal reconstruction with separate approaches offers acceptable cosmetic and func-tional outcomes.[7] If the defect involves greater than 30% to 40% of the orbital rim or includes the malar eminence along with a total maxillec-tomy defect, ideally the orbital defect is recon-structed with a scapular osseocutaneous free flap.

FLAP SELECTION, DESIGN, AND HARVEST

The harvest of the fasciocutaneous forearm flap is well described, but there are several technical considerations that should be considered when using this flap for orbital reconstruction. The amount of fat overlying the brachioradialis muscle in the forearm is important because sufficient fat is necessary for optimal orbital volume restoration. The flap design should be positioned on the arm to maximize this fat compartment and this is often the determining factor for choosing which arm to use rather than considerations for the use of the nondominant hand. A superficial, subdermal elevation is performed to maximize volume of the reconstruction. The fat should be connected to the vascular pedicle as much as possible to main-tain significant vascularity and should not be disconnected for a distance greater than 10 cm. The authors prefer to roll the fat snugly and suture it into position within the orbit rather than packing the fat to prevent postoperative settling of the volume restoration of the orbit. The more proximal

fat (but most distal from the vascular pedicle) should be in the external part of the roll, and the better vascularized, more distal fat, should be on the internal part of the roll. The roll or "cone" is oriented in the orbit with the distal forearm skin covering the fat, much like appearance of an ice-cream cone.

If a small amount of bone is needed for recon-structing the orbital rim (typically less than 30%–40%), a portion of the distal radius can be used along with the traditional radial forearm fasciocu-taneous flap.[6,7] When harvesting the bone for an osseocutaneous forearm flap, one must consider what the ultimate position of bone relative to the skin paddle will be in the final inset because there is much less mobility of the skin and bone, unlike the scapular osseocutaneous flap. This observa-tion also means that the flap inset rather than the patient's nondominant hand dictates the donor arm. The skin paddle tends to be trapezoidal with the longer side of the trapezoid running ante-riorly from just below the malar eminence to the postsuperomedial aspect of the resection that will cover the radial bone and the exposed native bone of the ascending process of the maxilla. The method of harvesting the radial bone is also critical. When harvesting an osseocutaneous fore-arm flap, a wedge of bone is removed that is centered on the attachment of the flexor retinac-ulum and the vascular supply from the radial artery. A wedge of bone less than 40% of the diameter of the radius rather than a traditional tangential cut allows for a more controlled harvest and probably more stability of the remaining bone. The cuts are made with a 5-mm, rounded-tip sagittal oscillating saw. Full-arm casting for 4 weeks is followed by 2 additional weeks of forearm casting to allow gradual loading and reorientation of the stress lines to minimize the risk of pathologic radius fracture. Alternatively, the radius can be plated with either a dynamic or limited-contact dynamic compression plate and plaster forearm splint for 7 days rather than prolonged casting.[22,23]

When larger amounts of bone are required (ie, greater than 40% of the rim, the malar eminence, or supraorbital bar), the osseocutaneous scapula flap is used.[6] One of the greatest advantages of the osseocutaneous scapula flap is the amount of tissue that can be harvested and the mobility of the soft tissue in relation to the bone harvest. In addition, the osseocutaneous scapula flap can be combined with the latissimus dorsi myocutaneous flap to resurface large, complicated three-dimen-sional defects. For the osseocutaneous scapula flap, the length of bone is maximized by making the superior osteotomy cut just below the inferior lip of the glenohumeral joint (approximately 1 cm below the joint) and taking the bone cut inferiorly to include the scapula tip. Unlike the iliac crest osseocutaneous flap, pedicle lengths of up to 15 cm can be obtained by dividing the subscapular vessels at the axillary artery and vein, obviating the need for vein grafts in many instances.

CASE EXAMPLES
Case 1

D.A. is 76-year-old man with a several year history of a 7-cm enlarging, ulcerative mass of the right cheek with extension to the right infraorbital region (**Fig. 1**A, B). Biopsy of the lesion revealed moderately differentiated squamous cell carcinoma. CT evaluation did indicate extension of the tumor into the orbit but the patient was found to have no enlarged lymph nodes on physical examination or radiologic evaluation. The patient underwent radical excision of the lesion, including all soft tissues overlying the face of the maxilla and the infraorbital rim (**Fig. 1**C). At surgery, the lateral and middle one third of the infraorbital rim was slightly eroded and this was removed at the time of surgery along with the contents of the right orbit. A large cervicofacial advancement flap with extension onto the neck was designed with the standing cutaneous deformity positioned at the melolabial fold to repair a defect that measured 8 × 9 cm. The standing deformity was not removed at the time of inset to preserve vascularity to the most distal portion of the flap. A small area in the preauricular region and the lateral nose was grafted with a full-thickness skin graft to prevent excessive tension on the local flap with closure. The most distal portion of the flap was sutured to the periosteum of the medial orbital rim. The orbital cavity was not skin grafted and was packed with half-inch gauge covered with bacitracin. The patient is now greater than 3 years from surgery with no recurrence and has continued to decline revision surgery to the standing cutaneous deformity of the medial cheek. The patient prefers to wear an eye patch rather than use an orbital prosthesis (**Fig. 2**).

Several points with regards to this case are worth mentioning in the ultimate decision of which reconstructive modality to use. Ipsilateral neck dissections typically require the sacrifice of the facial artery and cause a significant amount of disruption of the blood supply to large cervicofacial advancement flaps. The likelihood of flap necrosis would have been significantly higher had a neck dissection been performed and would have necessitated the use of a free flap in this clinical situation. Another important factor was the lack of concern with aesthetics by the patient. The patient was willing to except a suboptimal cosmetic result to shorten his hospital stay and not be concerned with the remote possibility of donor site morbidity or vascular compromise of a free tissue transfer (albeit with the possibility of necrosis of a large cervicofacial advancement flap). In addition, tumor surveillance was aided by the ability directly to visualize the exenteration cavity without the need for radiographic studies often required in a closed orbital reconstruction.

Case 2

K.D. is a 35-year-old man with a myxoid fibrosarcoma of the right maxillary sinus. He underwent a maxillectomy with the creation of a defect that included the entire infraorbital rim; the anterior, medial, and lateral buttresses of the maxilla; the lateral palate; and lateral alveolus. At the time of surgery, the periorbita of the right eye was not involved with tumor, but the entire inferior supporting structure of the orbit was removed including the orbital floor. The defect was reconstructed by placing a 10-hole 1.7-mm Leibinger mini-plate to span the infraorbital defect (**Fig. 3**A, B). An osseocutaneous radial forearm free flap was harvested from the left arm that measured 22 cm². The bone was osteotomized once to fit the contour of the plate and was secured to the plate. A Medpore implant was fashioned that was approximately 2-cm wide and 1.7-cm long and this slid under the eye and sutured anteriorly into place with three #4-0 Prolene sutures, which were passed through drill holes made in the bone. Care was taken to ensure that the prosthesis engaged the edge of bone along the resected orbital floor. Once this had been done, the cutaneous portion of the flap was sewn in place, facing in toward the oral cavity. This was sewn as high as possible in the defect to allow for fit of the obturator and obliteration of any potential space between the orbital floor reconstruction and the flap. More medially, the flap was tacked up to the root of the middle turbinate and to the septum more posteriorly. Laterally, it was tacked to residual pterygoid musculature. The pedicle was left open in the posterior aspect of the oral cavity along the cut edge of the buccal mucosa adjacent to the retromolar trigone. The pedicle was passed into the facial tunnel and down into the right neck.

This case example illustrates the use of an osseocutaneous radial forearm free flap for a defect that does not include an orbital exenteration, but where much of the supporting structure of the eye has been removed (**Fig. 3**C, D). In the authors' experience, patients who require postoperative radiotherapy have fewer problems with plate exposure when vascularized bone is used in the

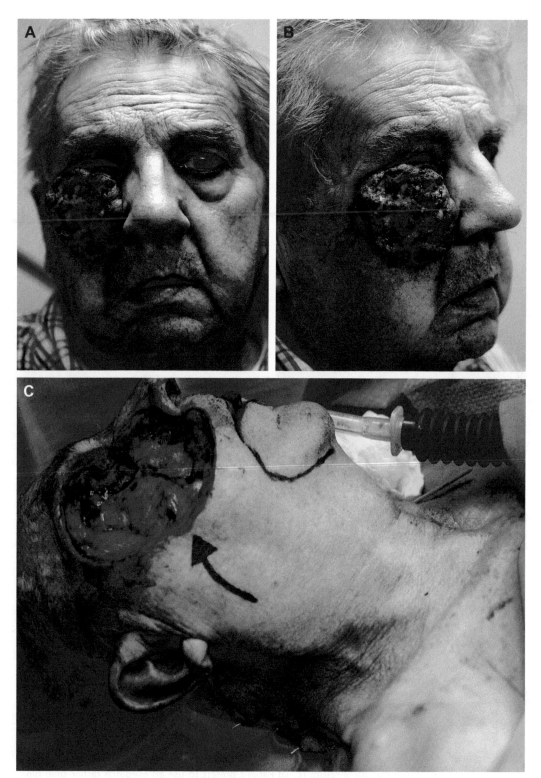

Fig. 1. Squamous cell carcinoma involving the right cheek and orbit reconstructed with local flap. The exenteration cavity was allowed to granulate and remained open. Preoperative frontal (*A*) and oblique (*B*) views. (*C*) Tumor excision and design of a large cervicofacial advancement flap for closure of the defect.

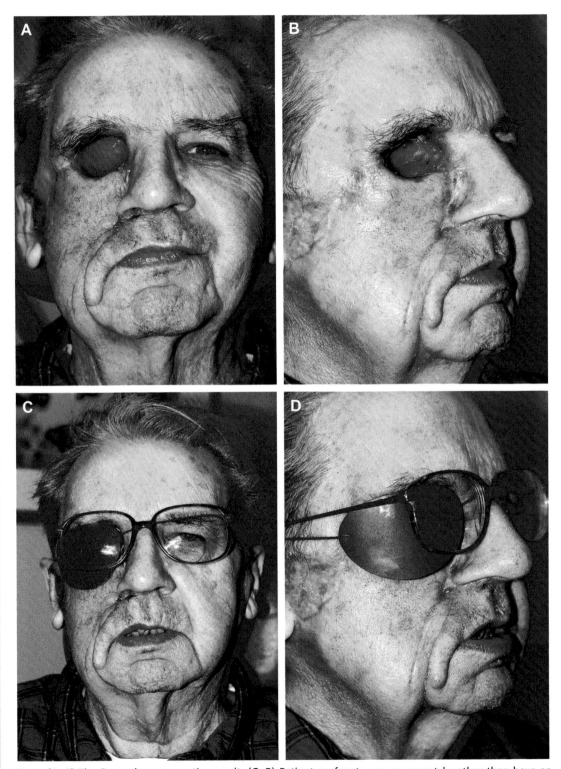

Fig. 2. (*A, B*) The 6-month postoperative result. (*C, D*) Patient prefers to use an eyepatch rather than have an orbital prosthesis fitted. Note the standing cutaneous deformity near the right melolabial fold. This was not removed at the time of the elevation of the local flap to prevent excessive narrowing of the flap at its base. The patient did not wish to have a second surgery to have this removed.

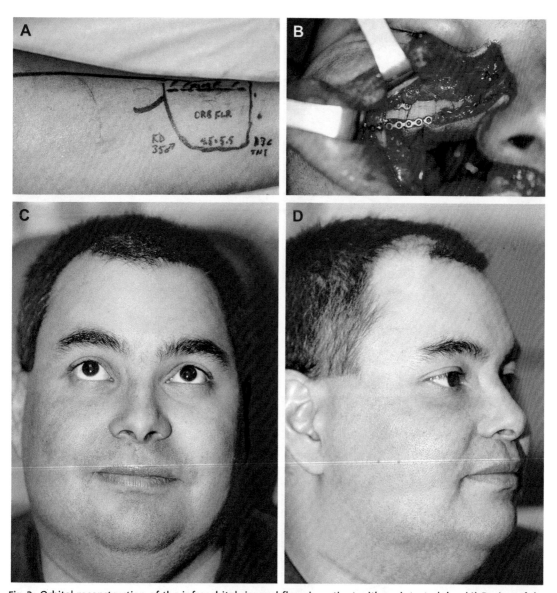

Fig. 3. Orbital reconstruction of the infraorbital rim and floor in patient with an intact globe. (*A*) Design of the osseocutaneous radial forearm free flap on the left forearm depicting location of rim and floor reconstruction. (*B*) Inset of osseocutaneous radial forearm free flap along inferior orbital rim with skin paddle supporting the orbital floor. (*C, D*) Two-year postoperative photographs. (*From* Chepeha DB, Moyer JS, Bradford CR, et al. Osseocutaneous radial forearm free tissue transfer for repair of complex midfacial defects. Arch Otolaryngol Head Neck Surg 2005;131:513–7; with permission.)

reconstruction. Regions of the maxillofacial skeleton that are convex, such as the infraorbital rim, are at a higher risk of plate extrusion given the thin skin and topographic prominence. Concentrating on the orbital reconstruction and preventing dystopia, diplopia, enophthalmos, ectropion, and other ocular complications is crucial to a successful outcome when the globe is maintained after tumor extirpation. The palatal defect is rehabilitated with an obturator and this generates functional outcomes similar to an intact palate,[7]

assuming appropriate anterolateral dentition remains to stabilize the prosthesis.

Case 3

M.M. is a 66-year-old woman with a remote history of radiation to the scalp with a 10 × 7 cm ulcerative lesion of the forehead that had been present for at least 7 years (**Fig. 4**A, B). There was obvious erosion of the frontal bar on clinical examination along with evidence of intraorbital and dural

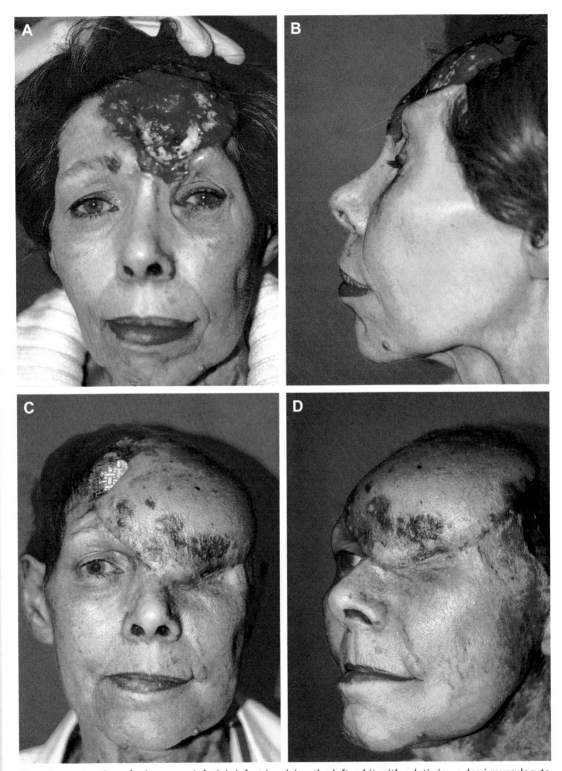

Fig. 4. Reconstruction of a large craniofacial defect involving the left orbit with a latissimus dorsi musculocutaneous free flap. (*A, B*) Preoperative view of an extensive basal cell carcinoma of the forehead invading the left orbit. (*C, D*) The 6-month postoperative view. Note the exposed mesh that occurred after completion of radiation with the loss of native scalp skin.

invasion on MRI. Pathology revealed aggressive growth pattern basal cell carcinoma. The patient underwent anterior craniofacial resection including the left orbital contents, 225 cm² of skin and scalp, 70 cm² of dura, and 90 cm² of calvarial bone including the frontal bar from left mid-orbit to glabella. The dura was repaired with Durepair and the craniectomy and frontal bar defect were reconstructed with 1.7-mm titanium mesh and hydroxyapatite cement. A left latissimus dorsi myocutaneous free tissue flap was harvested that included 225 cm² of skin and portions of the muscle

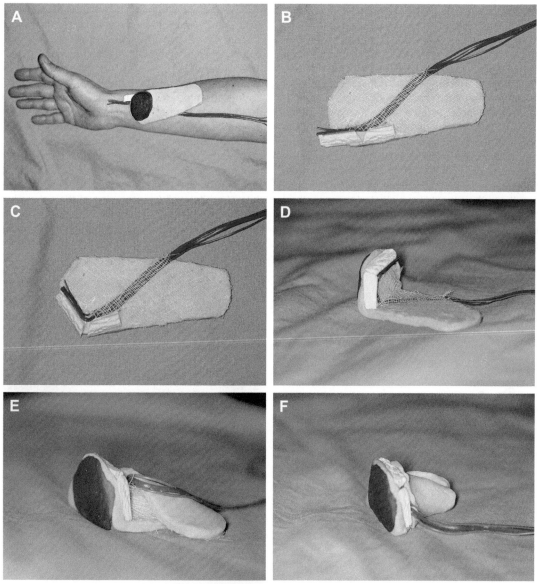

Fig. 5. Template and design of the osseocutaneous forearm flap on the right forearm. (A) The blue portion of the skin is harvested for the eyelids of the orbital subunit, the yellow portion is the subcutaneous fat, and the white portion is the radial bone. The flap is positioned at an angle so that the pedicle exits at a location that is optimal for the pedicle to be positioned at the inferior lateral orbital rim. The fat is thick over the brachioradialis muscle and is used preferentially for augmentation. (B–F) The bone is osteotomized and the flap is folded to allow the skin paddle to face forward such that the bone is positioned to recontour the lateral supraorbital rim and the lateral rim. The fat from the brachioradialis fat pad is folded toward the lateral aspect of the defect. The wrapped subcutaneous tissue is sutured into the position of a cone with monofilament suture. (From Chepeha DB, Wang SJ, Marentette LJ, et al. Restoration of the orbital aesthetic subunit in complex midface defects. Laryngoscope 2004;114:1706–13; with permission.)

were used to fill the orbital defect and reinforce the dural repair. Postoperatively, the patient underwent directed adjuvant radiotherapy to 40 Gy of the peripheral margins of the resection (**Fig.** 4C, D).

M.M. represents a large craniofacial defect with a communication between the orbit, sinuses, and intracranial contents. In addition to the need for the effective separation of intracranial and extracranial contents, there was a significant soft tissue defect that needed to be addressed to achieve a successful functional and aesthetic outcome. The orbital defect extended from the mid left orbit to the midline and it was believed that the addition of vascularized bone would not offer significant advantage to either cosmesis or function considering that most of the left orbital rim was still intact. In particular, the junction between the frontal bar and lateral orbital rim remained intact, preserving the appropriate geometry of this aesthetically important region. If the defect had extended more laterally to involve the entirety of the right frontal bar, the authors would have elected to reconstruct the defect with vascularized bone from the scapula in addition to the soft tissue from the latissimus dorsi free flap. In contrast, the thickness of the skin,

soft tissues, and muscle of the latissimus dorsi free flap offers significant protection to the titanium mesh repair in this region. The muscle portion of the flap was also placed within the orbital defect both to augment the tissue in this region and to protect the dural closure.

Case 4

D.O. is a 30-year-old woman with a several month history of left eye irritation and ptosis and was found to have a mass in the left lacrimal gland. She underwent excision of the lacrimal gland at an outside hospital and pathology revealed cribriform-pattern adenoid cystic carcinoma extending to the margins of the resection. She was referred to the University of Michigan for definitive resection and underwent a left orbital cranial approach to the orbit with orbital exenteration. The resection included the contents of the orbit; the lateral half of the supraorbital rim; the lateral orbital rim; the lateral orbital wall (greater wing of the sphenoid); and skin of the upper eyelid. The lower eyelid skin was preserved along with portion of the upper eyelid skin. A left osseocutaneous radial forearm

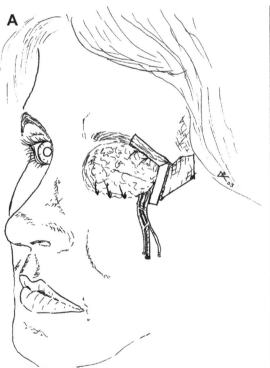 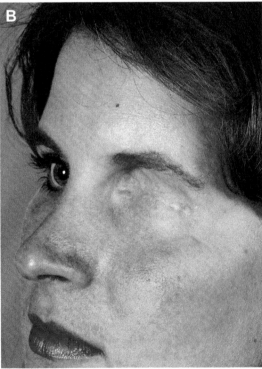

Fig. 6. Reconstruction of a left orbital exenteration cavity with an osseocutaneous radial forearm free flap. (*A*) The cone (fat) is slid back into the orbit, and the bone is plated with 1.7-mm miniplates to re-establish the superior and lateral orbital rim. The pedicle exits the orbit inferolaterally and split-calvarial bone grafts are used to repair the lateral orbital wall to maintain proper orbital volume. (*B*) Four-year postoperative result after revision surgery 2 years after initial reconstruction.

free flap was harvested, which included 15 cm^2 of skin, 35 cm^2 of fat, and 7 cm of radial bone (**Fig. 5**). The radial bone was used to reconstruct the lateral supraorbital rim and the entirety of the lateral orbital rim (**Fig. 6**). The radial bone was osteotomized once and the radial osteotomy site was stabilized with a 1.7-mm double-Y plate. The radial bone was attached in situ with two four-hole 1.7-mm miniplates. The lateral wall was reconstructed with a split-calvarial bone graft attached to the skull with 1.7-mm miniplates. The fat was used to fill the orbital defect and the cutaneous portion of the flap was used to replace the small skin defect of the left eyelid skin.

D.O. illustrates the use of an osteocutaneous radial forearm flap for the reconstruction of the supraorbital and lateral orbital rim that involved less than 40% of the orbital rim. The use of bone in the reconstruction is crucial for the maintenance

of facial contours. The use of vascularized bone in areas of facial prominence allows the surgeon to maintain thin skin over these aesthetically important areas and decrease the risk of either plate or bone exposure. Calvarial bone grafts have a greater degree of resorption, particularly after adjuvant radiotherapy.

This case also illustrates the benefits of preserving the eyelids in select cases to facilitate the repair of the orbit. The thin, pliable skin of the eyelids can then be used to resurface the closed orbit after excising the forearm skin paddle during subsequent revision surgery (see **Fig. 6**). This allows for a much more natural appearance to the reconstruction.

Case 5

D.W. is a 35-year-old man with a several month history of an expanding maxillary sinus mass that

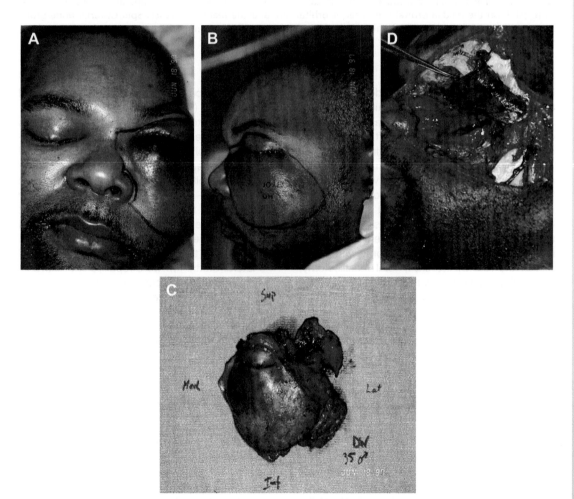

Fig. 7. Reconstruction of large orbitomaxillary defect with an osseocutaneous scapula free tissue flap. The defect involved the medial, lateral, and inferior orbital rims along with the malar eminence. (*A, B*) Preoperative views of patient with a left maxillary sinus squamous cell carcinoma. (*C*) Surgical specimen involving the left orbit and facial skin. (*D*) Postsurgical defect involving large portion of the left midface and orbit.

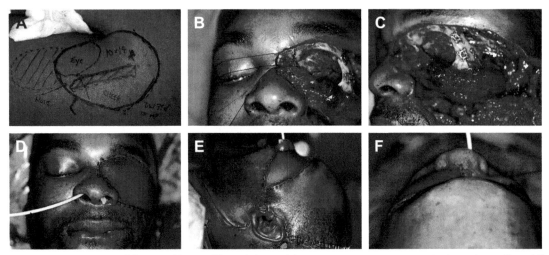

Fig. 8. Reconstruction of large orbitomaxillary defect with an osseocutaneous scapula free tissue flap. (*A*) Template of a left osseocutaneous free flap depicting the planned used of skin for the eye and cheek along with the lateral border of the scapula for the orbital rim and malar eminence. (*B, C*) Scapular bone has been inset to re-establish the medial orbital rim, inferior orbital rim, and the malar eminence. Split-calvarial bone grafts have been used for the lateral orbital rim and lateral orbital wall. (*D–F*) Immediate postoperative result of the reconstruction.

initially began as a small, reddened swelling beneath his left eye. He complains of diplopia and numbness of the left cheek and lip. Clinical examination reveals a large left cheek mass measuring 10 × 9 cm resulting in proptosis of the left eye (**Fig. 7**A, B). CT scan demonstrates a large left maxillary sinus mass with erosion of the orbital floor and anterior wall of the maxillary sinus with extension into the soft tissues of the cheek and posterior orbit. There is bilateral neck adenopathy. The patient underwent craniofacial resection including frontal craniotomy with resection of the roof of the orbit, total maxillectomy, and orbital exenteration with removal of the lateral orbit and malar eminence (**Fig. 7**C, D). The cutaneous excision measured 10 × 14 cm. The floor of the anterior cranial fossa was repaired with a pericranial flap that extended back to the planum sphenoidale under the frontal lobe. An osseocutaneous free scapular transfer was harvested to repair the malar eminence, inferior orbital rim, medial orbital rim, and the large cutaneous defect that was created by the resection. The entire lateral border of the scapula was removed, which measured approximately 10 cm. A tab of fat measuring 8 × 6 cm was harvested from the inferior periscapular portion of the scapular flap to fill the orbit and reinforce the dural closure and 10 × 14 cm of skin was harvested to reconstruct the cutaneous defect. The lateral orbital rim was repaired with split calvarial bone grafts using 1.7-mm miniplates to affix the grafts to the supraorbital

bar and the scapular bone of the inferior orbital reconstruction (**Fig. 8**).

D.W. illustrates the use of the osseocutaneous free flap for the repair of large craniofacial resections that involves both an important functional component (separation and reinforcement of the dural and orbital reconstruction) and cosmetic component (re-establishment of the facial contour and closure of the cutaneous defect). The defect involved greater than 40% of the orbital rim and consisted of the lateral, inferior, and medial orbital rim along with the malar eminence. Portions of the lateral orbital rim were repaired with calvarial bone, but this was securely positioned under the soft tissue portion of the flap. The osseocutaneous free flap is perhaps the best flap choice for defects of the orbitomaxillary complex that require bone and large amounts of soft tissue.

SUMMARY

Large paranasal and skull base tumors requiring orbital exenteration for tumor clearance frequently involves an extensive resection of the soft tissues and bony architecture of the orbitomaxillary complex. Defects of this region often create a communication between the intracranial and extracranial contents that must be repaired to prevent postoperative complications. In addition to the functional requirements of the reconstruction, the resection of large areas of bone and soft tissue pose a demanding challenge for the aesthetic reconstruction of the region. Unlike local and regional tissues, free tissue transfer can reliably separate the extracranial and intracranial compartments and restore the bony and soft tissue architecture of the obitomaxillary complex.

REFERENCES

1. Nassab RS, Thomas SS, Murray D. Orbital exenteration for advanced periorbital skin cancers: 20 years experience. J Plast Reconstr Aesthet Surg 2007;60:1103–9.
2. Tyers AG. Orbital exenteration for invasive skin tumours. Eye 2006;20:1165–70.
3. Ben Simon GJ, Schwarcz RM, Douglas R, et al. Orbital exenteration: one size does not fit all. [see comment]. Am J Ophthalmol 2005;139:11–7.
4. Gunalp I, Gunduz K, Duruk K. Orbital exenteration: a review of 429 cases. Int Ophthalmol 1995;19:177–84.
5. Moyer JS, Chepeha DB, Teknos TN. Contemporary skull base reconstruction. Curr Opin Otolaryngol Head Neck Surg 2004;12:294–9.
6. Chepeha DB, Wang SJ, Marentette LJ, et al. Restoration of the orbital aesthetic subunit in complex midface defects. Laryngoscope 2004;114:1706–13.
7. Chepeha DB, Moyer JS, Bradford CR, et al. Osseocutaneous radial forearm free tissue transfer for repair of complex midfacial defects. Arch Otolaryngol Head Neck Surg 2005;131:513–7.
8. Ketcham AS, Hoye RC, Van Buren JM, et al. Complications of intracranial facial resection for tumors of the paranasal sinuses. Am J Surg 1966;112:591–6.
9. Ketcham AS, Wilkins RH, Vanburen JM, et al. A combined intracranial facial approach to the paranasal sinuses. Am J Surg 1963;106:698–703.
10. Johns ME, Winn HR, McLean WC, et al. Pericranial flap for the closure of defects of craniofacial resection. Laryngoscope 1981;91:952–9.
11. Snyderman CH, Janecka IP, Sekhar LN, et al. Anterior cranial base reconstruction: role of galeal and pericranial flaps. Laryngoscope 1990;100:607–14.
12. Jackson IT, Adham MN, Marsh WR. Use of the galeal frontalis myofascial flap in craniofacial surgery. Plast Reconstr Surg 1986;77:905–10.
13. Cordeiro PG, Santamaria E. A classification system and algorithm for reconstruction of maxillectomy and midfacial defects. Plast Reconstr Surg 2000; 105:2331–46 [discussion: 47–8].
14. Cordeiro PG, Santamaria E, Kraus DH, et al. Reconstruction of total maxillectomy defects with preservation of the orbital contents. Plast Reconstr Surg 1998;102:1874–84 [discussion: 85–7].
15. Granick MS, Ramasastry SS, Newton ED, et al. Reconstruction of complex maxillectomy defects with the scapular-free flap. Head Neck 1990;12: 377–85.
16. Swartz WM, Banis JC, Newton ED, et al. The osteocutaneous scapular flap for mandibular and maxillary reconstruction. Plast Reconstr Surg 1986;77: 530–45.
17. Brown JS. Deep circumflex iliac artery free flap with internal oblique muscle as a new method of immediate reconstruction of maxillectomy defect. Head & Neck 1996;18:412–21.
18. Brown JS, Rogers SN, McNally DN, et al. A modified classification for the maxillectomy defect. Head & Neck 2000;22:17–26.
19. Anthony JP, Foster RD, Sharma AB, et al. Reconstruction of a complex midfacial defect with the folded fibular free flap and osseointegrated implants. Ann Plast Surg 1996;37:204–10.
20. Futran ND, Wadsworth JT, Villaret D, et al. Midface reconstruction with the fibula free flap. Arch Otolaryngol Head Neck Surg 2002;128:161–6.
21. Triana RJ Jr, Uglesic V, Virag M, et al. Microvascular free flap reconstructive options in patients with partial and total maxillectomy defects. Arch Facial Plast Surg 2000;2:91–101.
22. Waits CA, Toby EB, Girod DA, et al. Osteocutaneous radial forearm free flap: long-term radiographic evaluation of donor site morbidity after prophylactic plating of radius. J Reconstr Microsurg 2007;23: 367–72.
23. Werle AH, Tsue TT, Toby EB, et al. Osteocutaneous radial forearm free flap: its use without significant donor site morbidity. Otolaryngol Head Neck Surg 2000;123:711–7.

Maxillofacial Trauma Reconstruction

Neal D. Futran, MD, DMD

KEYWORDS

• Maxillofacial • Free flap • Mandible • Midface
• Rigid fixation • Facial reconstruction • Trauma

Advances in many areas of surgery and medicine have shaped the contemporary management of facial trauma patients. Current management reflects the evolution of both bony and soft tissue reconstruction principles and techniques. External splinting to hold fracture fragments in position and interfragmentary wiring of facial fractures were routinely used through the 1970s.[1] These techniques used minimal exposure of bony anatomy and relied heavily on closed reduction and wire suspension techniques.[2,3] In the mid-1980s a number of conceptual, surgical, and biomaterial advances ushered in the current era of facial fracture management. The concept and importance of facial buttresses in the functional and aesthetic reconstruction of the face were recognized.[4–6] CT scanning of facial injuries became incorporated as an essential component in the contemporary diagnostic work-up.[7] Plate and screw technology, which allowed rigid fixation of fracture fragments, and bone grafts became routine.[8,9] In addition to allowing rigid fixation of bone fragments, the use of plates and screws facilitated complicated reconstructions by decreasing the number and complexity of bone grafts required as batons to stabilize fracture fragments.[9] Plate and screw technology has continued to evolve from poorly malleable, high profile, adaptive stainless steel plates to very low profile osseointegrating titanium plates, and the use of locking screw mandibular reconstruction systems.[10] The locking screw mandibular reconstruction plates have greatly facilitated both interim and permanent mandibular reconstruction, and have largely replaced external fixation devices in the acute mandibular trauma patient with segmental bone loss. With the increased sophistication of the internal bony repairs, the development of cosmetically acceptable, extended-access approaches to the underlying facial skeleton was required.

Paralleling these advances, the last several decades have seen an exponential growth in the variety and sophistication of procedures available for importing tissue into the head and neck region for reconstructive purposes. Limited tissue volume, poor adaptability to complex defects, multiple stages, and the modest vascular supply of local cutaneous and walking-tube type flaps have limited their use in major defect reconstruction to the final cosmetic stages, in which relatively minor contouring is needed.[11] With these flaps, significant volumes of soft tissue could be mobilized. Length limitations of the vascular pedicle, unreliability of bone transfer, and poor contourability of these relatively bulky flaps into complex and often composite defects, however, remained problematic. Free tissue transfer has made it possible to bring well-vascularized bone and soft tissue into a hostile wound environment with excellent survival of the flap tissues or free-bone grafts invested by the vascularized flap.[12] This has allowed for simultaneous reconstruction of the bony facial skeleton and the overlying soft tissue soon after injury. With this reconstructive technique there has been a shift away from delayed bony and soft tissue reconstruction toward definitive reconstruction as soon as possible following injury to minimize the scar contracture of the facial soft tissues.[13–16] Although there are indications for all of these techniques, free tissue transfer has dramatically expanded the armamentarium of the reconstructive surgeon. The reconstructive flap best suited to address the wound

Department of Otolaryngology-Head and Neck Surgery, University of Washington, 1959 NE Pacific Street, Box 356515, Seattle, WA 98195, USA
E-mail address: nfutran@u.washington.edu

Facial Plast Surg Clin N Am 17 (2009) 239–251
doi:10.1016/j.fsc.2009.01.003
1064-7406/09/$ – see front matter © 2009 Elsevier Inc. All rights reserved.

environment and the functional and aesthetic problems of the defect may be chosen from an extensive array of flap designs and standard flap modifications.[17,18]

Gunshot wounds and avulsive trauma to the face have added new dimensions to the complexity of defects confronting the facial reconstructive surgeon. The essential difference between most blunt facial injuries and ballistic or avulsive facial injuries is the severity of the soft and hard tissue loss or damage. An evolving pattern of tissue loss is also observed. Tissue necrosis and infection from hematoma, dead space, and ischemia comprise and complicate attempts at definitive primary repair.[19,20] Application of modern principles of fracture management and wound care, however, allows restoration of the facial framework until a healthy tissue bed is achieved for definitive repair.

A staged approach to the reconstruction of the severe facial trauma patient is recommended (**Box 1**).[21] Having a checklist of goals to be accomplished in a phased fashion allows a systematic and ordered approach to these patients to prevent an oversight of important steps in both the facial and systemic trauma treatment. The management of these patients can be broken into three phases defined by specific reconstructive, rehabilitative, and global patient management goals. The phases are not defined by temporal units and may be proceeded through rapidly or may require more time at a particular phase so that all of the goals of that phase are met.

PHASE I: THE INITIAL ENCOUNTER

Discipline is required when faced with a devastating facial injury to ensure that the ABCs of trauma management are undertaken in the emergency room. The airway is secured, the patient's breathing is stabilized, bleeding is controlled with direct pressure, and the cervical spine is cleared. If multisystem trauma is evident, all of the systemic injuries should be evaluated by the appropriate services before moving the patient from the emergency room to the operating room for initial management of the facial wound. The incidence of major vascular injury in facial gunshot wounds is 10% to 50%, depending on the entry site, and this possibility should be carefully evaluated with an angiogram or CT angiogram. The indications for angiographic evaluation can be found in a number of excellent papers.[22–26] Many of these injuries involve intracranial or ocular trauma,[27–30] and an early involvement of the ophthalmologist and neurosurgeon facilitates getting the patient to the operating room quickly. An accurate visual

evaluation is crucial in shaping the management of the patient. The visual status of the eyes (or remaining eye, if one is obviously nonfunctional) is crucial information to have before the first trip to the operating room. If open intracranial injuries are present, neurosurgical management figures

---

Box 1
The three phases of reconstruction after major gunshot wounds and avulsive trauma

Phase I: The initial encounter

1. The ABCs of trauma management
2. Initial operating room management

   a. Management of intracranial, ocular, and other life- or limb-threatening injuries
   b. Establishment of occlusal relationships
   c. Debridement of foreign material and obviously nonviable tissue
   d. Stenting of the facial soft tissue envelope

      Definitive free-bone graft reconstruction in areas with adequate soft tissue coverage

      Interim bone graft reconstruction in areas with unsatisfactory soft tissue coverage

      Reconstruction plate fixation of segmental mandibular defects

   e. Best possible soft tissue closure
3. Planning of definitive bony and soft tissue reconstruction
4. Planning of dental and facial prosthetic rehabilitation in conjunction with flap selection
5. Psychiatric and social service evaluation

Phase II: The definitive reconstruction

1. Free tissue transfer procedure

   a. Reconstruction of major mandibular and maxillary defects
   b. Satisfactory soft tissue coverage of all underlying bone, internal, and external defects
2. Importation of adequate soft tissue to allow cosmetic contouring
3. Free-bone graft reconstruction of upper face, nasal profile, and periorbital area

Phase III: Aesthetic and functional refinement

1. Major flap debulking and contouring as required
2. Dental rehabilitation with tissue-borne, implant-retained, or implant-borne dental prostheses
3. Final oral commissuroplasty
4. Adjunctive cosmetic measures

prominently into the planning of the first procedure.

Traumatic defects are created by high-energy instruments of destruction outside the operating room. Shards of glass and steel or bullets do not create defects with a respect for vital structures or tissue planes. The wound is created in a dirty environment without the benefit of preoperative antibiotics. Bone is shattered and soft tissues are torn and avulsed or destroyed. Severe facial trauma defects present with a variety of different structural peculiarities that the surgeon needs to explore and understand. The degree of bone and soft tissue destruction and avulsion is an unknown when the surgeon enters the operating room for the first time with a severe trauma patient.

If the injury is caused by ballistic injury, special considerations are warranted. Bullets are not sterile, and inoculate the wound with fragments of clothing or any other substance that they pass through before entering the body, including skin bacteria.[31] The defect may be contaminated with orosinonasal secretions or foreign material, and frequently contains nonviable soft tissue and bone. The incidence of wound healing complications from even low-energy gunshot wounds that traverse the oral cavity is 39%,[30] and an infection rate of 100% following close range shotgun injuries to the face has been reported.[24] Gunshot wounds involving a surrounding rim of devitalized tissue become infected rapidly by two mechanisms:[32] primary infection resulting from inoculation of infecting bacteria by the bullet, and secondary infection resulting from contamination of the wound once it has been made.

In animal experiments, prompt institution of antibiotics has been demonstrated to reduce the bacterial concentration of the wound if debridement is delayed for up to 12 hours. The volume of necrotic tissue requiring debridement is decreased the sooner the debridement is done following injury, and if the experimental animal has been treated with antibiotics.[33]

Bacterial count is also related to the degree of tissue destruction, with higher-energy wounds resulting in greater bacterial counts at early (6 hour) debridement.[32] These studies point out the importance of early initial debridement of necrotic tissues from severe facial injuries and the importance of beginning antibiotic treatment as soon as possible. This aspect of facial trauma, particularly following gunshot wounds, previously dictated that reconstruction begin with soft tissue closure, despite underlying bone loss. Only after complete soft tissue healing occurred could the underlying bone loss be reconstructed in a sterile wound.[12,19] The scar contracture that formed

during the soft tissue healing in these wounds frequently rendered an optimal final bony and soft tissue repair impossible. With regard to this critically important aspect of facial reconstruction, free tissue transfer has dramatically advanced the management of the severe open facial trauma patient.[12,21,34]

Once the patient is stabilized and cleared for general anesthetic, the initial operative management should take place as soon as possible. The goals of the initial procedure are to address intracranial injuries, debride all foreign material and obviously nonviable tissue, establish and stabilize occlusal relationships in remaining tooth-bearing segments, and perform satisfactory bony reconstruction to maintain the facial soft tissue envelope. During wound debridement, if there is a question about the viability of tissue, it is retained to declare itself within 24 to 72 hours. This is particularly true of skin margins and the tissues of the nose, palate, lips, and medial canthal areas where the survival of tissues may significantly influence the choice of flap reconstruction or how a particular flap is used for definitive reconstruction.

In most cases, occlusion can be established acutely with maxillomandibular fixation. In cases with significant or palatal or mandibular comminution, the acute fabrication of dental splints may serve to minimize lingual rotation of mandibular segments when maxillomandibular fixation is applied, assist in establishing the horizontal arch dimension, assist in fracture stabilization, and function as a tension band.[35]

If a craniotomy for management of an intracranial injury is required, this should be performed initially. Obliteration or cranialization of the frontal sinus, if required, should take place at this initial procedure.[12] If reconstructed with free-bone grafts following management of frontal sinus, bone grafts can be obtained from the inner table of the craniotomy bone while the neurosurgeons are working. If the anterior cranial fossa floor is disrupted, an extended pericranial flap should be harvested to assist in separating the sinonasal and intracranial spaces with vascularized tissue.[12,15] The harvest of this flap may extend posterior to the coronal incision if the incision is not extended down to bone. This permits the harvest of a very long flap. This flap is also useful to line the roof of a reconstructed orbit, or to invest upper facial bone grafts.

Every effort should be made at the initial surgery to perform enough underlying bone reconstruction to prevent contracture of the facial soft tissues.[6,12] This goal is addressed at the initial procedure in several ways: (1) definitive bone grafting in all areas with adequate soft tissue coverage; (2)

temporary bone grafting in areas with unsatisfactory soft tissue coverage for interim stenting of the surrounding soft tissues; and (3) locking reconstruction plate fixation of segmental mandibular defects with anticipated definitive bone reconstruction during phase II (**Fig. 1**).

The plate requires only a small amount of soft tissue for temporary coverage, and does not seem to incite problematic infections if it becomes exposed in the oral cavity for a short period of time in a patient on antibiotics. If the overlying and internal soft tissue trauma is minimal and sufficient soft tissue remains for complete coverage of the bone grafts, this initial bone reconstruction may be definitive. If insufficient soft tissue is available to cover the midfacial bone grafts definitively, the degree of bone and soft tissues should still be placed to keep the remaining soft tissues of the midface areas stented. In this case, the bone grafts are viewed as interim until the definitive procedure is performed, which allows reconstruction of both the underlying bone and surrounding soft tissues. Temporary bone grafts in the maxillary area tolerate exposure to the sinonasal tract, and internal plate exposure in this area is frequently not a severe problem (**Fig. 1A**). As long as the plate and bone grafts are stable, they may be left alone[12,19,20] and replaced at the time of the definitive reconstruction when adequate soft tissue coverage is available.

The best available soft tissue closure is used without significant distortion of the soft tissues. It must be kept in mind that the surgeon is returning soon during the definitive reconstruction, and rotation or advancement flaps performed to obtain skin closure should be done with an eye toward that procedure. The size of the oral stoma should not be compromised in any way to facilitate closure during this or the second phase. Access to the oral cavity for the placement of osseointegrated implants and dental and prosthetic work must be maintained. The remainder of phase I consists largely of a detailed planning of what will be performed at phase II. The extent of masticatory load-bearing bone lost from the mandible and maxilla, and the amount of internal and external soft tissue loss are now known. In trauma patients with otherwise normal health and anticipated life spans, bone reconstruction of segmental mandibular defects is preferred. This group of patients frequently has remaining dentition, and prolonged mastication of a normal unlimited diet without bone reconstruction results in eventual failure of mandibular reconstruction plate bridging a segmental defect. This is particular true for the anterior defects that make up most cases. The remaining dentition of the maxillary and mandibular arches should be carefully assessed in conjunction with a maxillofacial prosthodontist. A decision regarding the possible need for osseointegrated implants versus tissue-borne denture prosthesis for the mandible should be made. If it is clear that implants in the reconstructed mandible are required, the mandibular reconstruction should be planned accordingly, using a bone flap that permits the safe placement of osseointegrated implants.[36] In most cases this is the fibula, iliac crest, or scapula.[37]

The maxillary arch may be nearly entirely destroyed in severe midline facial trauma from self-inflicted submental shotgun wounds. In cases with significant loss of maxillary and palatal bone, the decision is whether a tissue-borne denture-obturator can be retained, supported, and stabilized in the defect to provide satisfactory palatal obruation and functional dental rehabilitation. In general, if greater than one half of the maxillary arch and hard palate are destroyed,

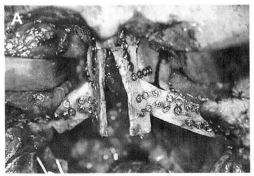
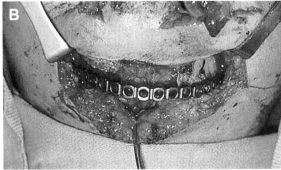

Fig. 1. (*A*) Cranial bone grafts are used at the primary surgical procedure to restore the naso-orbital complex and maintain the soft tissue envelope after an avulsive gunshot injury to the midface. (*B*) A locking reconstruction plate is placed at the primary surgical procedure to stabilize and maintain mandibular shape while bridging the defect created by a gunshot injury.

the use of a tissue-borne denture obturator is problematic. This is particularly true when significant losses of overlying soft tissue have occurred. In these cases, free-tissue transfer reconstruction of the maxillary arch with osseointegrated implant stabilization of denture prosthesis may be the only means of providing functional maxillary dental rehabilitiation.[31] In addition to the dental prosthetic rehabilitation, a detailed plan is needed for facial prosthetic rehabilitation of the nose or an ocular prosthesis if an enucleation has been performed.

Significant systemic injuries that potentially hinder return to the operating room for phase II should be managed as quickly as possible during this period. Finally, the provision of both psychiatric and social service consultation should be undertaken as necessary.

PHASE II: THE DEFINITIVE RECONSTRUCTION

Phase II reconstruction with free-tissue transfer allows the wounds to heal without infection and with as little scarring and contraction as possible. This process helps tissue to retain elasticity, and a better functional result can be expected.

The primary goals of the definitive reconstructive procedure, both of which are used for functional and aesthetic purposes in shaping the final result, are the reconstruction of the underlying bony framework and the provision of adequate soft tissue.

Free-tissue transfer has made it possible to bring well-vascularized bone and soft tissue into a hostile wound environment with excellent survival of the flap tissues or free-bone grafts invested by the vascularized flap.[21,34] This has allowed for simultaneous reconstruction of the bony facial skeleton and the overlying soft tissue soon after injury. With this reconstructive technique there has been a shift away from delayed bony reconstruction toward definitive reconstruction as soon as possible following injury to minimize the scar contracture of the facial soft tissue.[12,21,34]

With the incorporation of free tissue transfer into the management of severe facial trauma, current reconstruction guidelines should include (1) extended access and exposure of fractures; (2) rigid internal fixation of fractures, free-bone grafts, and vascularized flap bone; (3) reconstruction of the underlying bone concurrently with the overlying soft tissue during the definitive procedure, which should be performed as soon as reasonably possible following the injury; and (4) selection of a free-tissue transfer flap that maximizes the adjunctive reconstructive procedures.

The techniques of free-tissue transfer may also be used in the microvascular replantation of avulsed tissue from the head and neck, and the possibility of vascularized replantation should always be considered. Although there are a variety of situations in which microvascular transfer is used in severe facial trauma, most can be placed into one of the following groups: (1) replacement of deficient bone or soft tissue for aesthetic or functional purposes, (2) vascular coverage of underlying bone or other structures, or (3) microvascular replantation of avulsed tissue.

The use of vascularized bone to replace large segmental areas of mandible is currently preferred, and is often essential if the injury has destroyed or avulsed significant floor of mouth and chin soft tissue (**Fig. 2**). Vascularized bone provides a rapid, dependable reconstruction; may be inset with its own vascularized soft tissue coverage; and is capable of surviving in the contaminated environment of the floor of the mouth. At the time of bone flap insetting, the most expedient procedure is to secure the bone flap by lagging it onto the existing locking screw reconstruction plate (if one was placed in the initial procedure). A fresh bone cut on the native mandible should be performed 0.5 to 1 cm back from the jagged end of the bone, and maximal surface area contact between the flap and native mandible should be obtained. If a fibula flap is being used, an attempt to fixate the flap as high as possible on the native mandible should be made. This facilitates later dental rehabilitation by placing the denture or implant-bearing surface of the bone as close as possible to the height of the remaining alveolar crest. Although not the first choice for mandibular reconstruction based on the quality and quantity of bone stock available, the combined scapular osteocutaneous and latissimus dorsi free flap may be indicated for the importation of sufficient soft tissues to drape over midfacial bone grafts, provide internal and external lining, and reconstruct the mandible. The exceptions to vascularized bone reconstruction of the mandible are cases in which there is adequate remaining soft tissues overlying the mandible and large fragments of the mandible have remained attached to periosteum, which can be rigidly fixated. This occasionally is the case in submental gunshot injuries, and may be the result of the muzzle of the gun being placed under the chin, posterior to the arch of the mandible, or cases in which the bullet path is anterior to the midpoint of the mandible.

Frequently, in these cases soft tissue replacement is required both intraorally and in adjacent perioral areas externally. In many cases a portion of the flap paddle can be de-epithelialized and the remaining tissues of the lip essentially draped

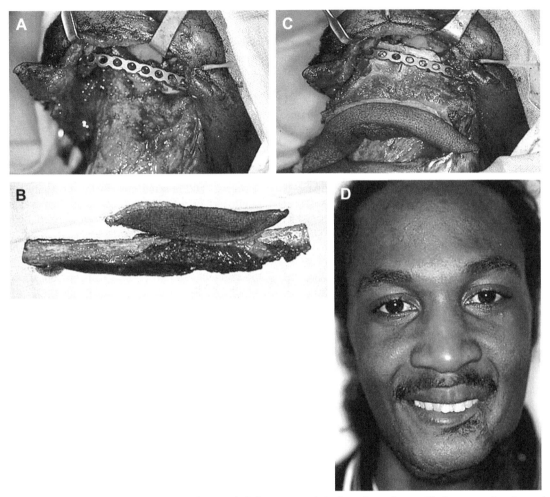

Fig. 2. (A) Mandibular reconstruction plate and defect exposed during phase II mandibular reconstruction of gunshot wound victim. (B) Fibula flap harvested. (C) Fibula flap osteotomized and secured in the defect with monocortical screws. The fibula soft tissue is rotated over the plate and recreates the floor of mouth tissues. (D) Patient 1 year after definitive reconstruction.

over and sutured to the de-epithelialized segment. This provides satisfactory soft tissue coverage, but does make initial restoration of the normal gingivo-labial and gingivolingual sulci anatomy difficult.

The reconstructive goals in the maxillary arch are to create a neoalveolar ridge of stable bone suitable as a prosthesis-bearing or implant-bearing surface and to close the palatal defect (Fig. 3). The surface of the surgically reconstructed maxillary arch is frequently flatter than the native maxillary alveolar arch and may function well as a stable prosthesis-bearing support surface to stabilize the denture against upward masticatory forces and prevent motion during function. Because of the blunted neoalveolar contours, however, the denture tends to fall away from the reconstructed roof of the mouth unless either

satisfactory dentition remains to serve as dental abutments or osseointegrated implants are used.

If over one half of the maxillary dental arch is destroyed, including significant losses of the nasomaxillary and zygomaticomaxillary bony buttresses and overlying central facial soft tissues, then a vascularized bone reconstruction of the maxillary dental arch likely is required to restore long-term function dental rehabilitation.

The factors influencing the approach to reconstruction in this area are suitability of the overall bone and soft tissue defect for tissue-born denture-obturator prosthetic rehabilitation without free-tissue transfer reconstruction, and need for overlying soft tissue reconstruction.

Residual dentition provides a definite advantage in the construction of tissue-borne dentures or

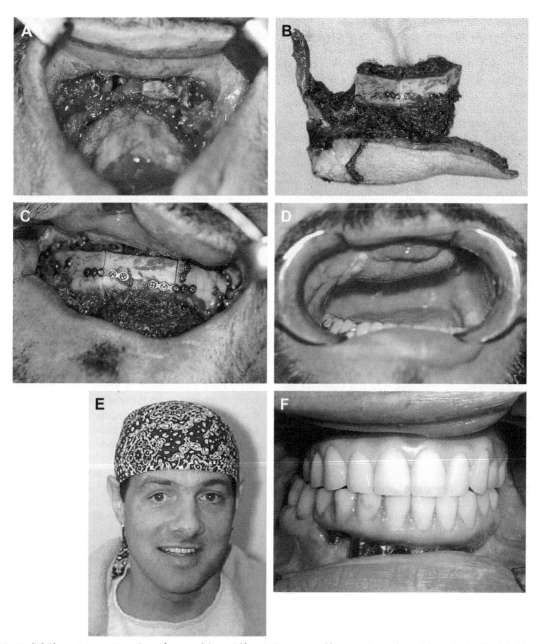

Fig. 3. (*A*) Phase II reconstruction of an avulsive midface injury caused by a motorcycle accident. Defect is debrided to healthy tissue. (*B*) Fibula flap osteotomized to recreate the maxilla. (*C*) Fibula flap secured to adjacent bone with 1.5-mm titanium miniplates. The fibula soft tissue recreates the palate. (*D*) Intraoral view 3 months after reconstruction just before osseointegrated implant placement. (*E*) Patient 1 year after reconstruction. (*F*) Intraoral view of osseointegrated implant-borne prosthesis 1 year after reconstruction.

denture-obturator prostheses for the patient with an extensive palatomaxillary defect. The dental abutments may be engaged with dental clasps on the prosthesis to assist in retention of the prosthesis against the forces of gravity, and to provide some stabilization during function. The semirigid stabilization of the dental clasps does not, however, prevent significant motion of the prosthesis during functional loading in extensive composite midfacial defects. In these cases, this type of rehabilitation may be satisfactory to provide cosmetic rehabilitation, but it does not address the functional problem of inadequate prosthesis support caused by limited prosthesis-bearing surface area within the defect. In a small percentage of patients, the placement of osseointegrated implants into the residual bone of the unreconstructed maxilla may be satisfactory to provide adequate retention of denture-obturator prosthesis. Successful use of implant-retained prosthesis in large maxillary defects, however, without surgical reconstruction of the underlying bone, is fraught with a number of problems. This technique should be limited to small defects.[38]

Surgical reconstruction of the maxillary arch replaces the defect with a stable prosthesis-bearing surface capable of distributing the support symmetrically over a large area. The reconstructive goals in these cases are to create a neoalveolar ridge of the stable bone suitable as a prosthesis-bearing or implant-bearing surface and to close the palatal defect.

The reconstruction should also provide replacement or support of facial soft tissues. The fibula osteofasciocutaneous flap has gained considerable popularity in mandibular reconstruction and has been reported for maxillary reconstruction (see **Fig. 3**).[39,40] It provides excellent bone stock for osseointegration and relatively thin skin paddle with a satisfactory orientation to the bone for intraoral soft tissue coverage of the reconstructed maxillary arch. The ability to fabricate zygomatico-maxillary buttresses and a neomaxillary arch from the fibula bone suggests that this flap is a satisfactory alternative to the scapula for maxillary arch reconstruction. The vascularized radial bone, although small in volume when compared with the bony free flaps, is an excellent choice to reconstruct the premaxillary segment or to augment mandibular bone stock in cases where bone has been lost, but there is no segmental loss. The scapula osteocutaneous flap has also been used for these reconstructions. The lateral border of the scapula provides adequate bone stock for osseointegration,[36,37] and the transversely oriented skin paddle is used to close over the bone intraorally. During harvest of the scapula bone, medial extensions of the scapula are harvested to serve as bony anchors and to recreate the curvature of the maxillary arch, and it is positioned inferiorly when the flap is inset. Bone plating and plating of the scapula to the remaining maxillary bone are done with 2-mm miniplates. The skin paddle is closed over the scapular bone intraorally and sutured to the posterior margin of the palatal defect. The scapular skin paddle may be folded along a de-epithelialized segment to allow for placement of some of the skin paddle on the nasal surface of the palatal reconstruction. An anterior extension of the skin paddle may be brought out anteriorly (under the lip as described previously)

to replace facial soft tissue. Remaining mucosa from the nose and maxillary sinuses can also be recruited to reline the nasal floor. Debulking of the scapular skin paddle and placement of implants, if not done primarily, may be done after an initial healing time of 6 to 8 weeks.

The bone of the periorbital area, forehead, and nasal dorsum bears no significant loads and has much sharper external contour angles than the bone of the mandible or maxillary arch. Free-bone grafts are easier to shape for restoration of the normal form in these areas than are most vascularized bone flaps and, if covered with healthy soft tissue, have excellent survival (see **Fig. 1A**).[35] Membranous cortical bone available with outer or inner table cranial bone grafts demonstrates excellent survival despite exposure to the sinonasal tract, and is readily available within the operative field.[41,42] In some cases a small area of exposed cranial bone graft within the sinonasal compartment is covered with granulation tissue and mucosa with only conservative antibiotic and rigorous hygiene. The relatively thick cortical bone from this site facilitates rigid fixation, which is crucial to graft take and survival. Rib is rarely used because of its lower-volume retention compared with cranial bone grafts. Cranial bone grafts retain structural integrity and rigid fixation for months, despite exposure to sinonasal contamination. In some cases, a small area of exposed cranial bone graft within the sinonasal compartment becomes covered with granulation tissue and eventually only mucosa with conservative antibiotic and rigorous hygiene management.

In anticipation of phase III, osseointegrated implants can be placed primarily into maxillary or mandibular reconstructions if it is certain that a tissue-borne denture is not satisfactory. In most cases, however, the changes in perioral anatomy that occur with healing are much greater than those encountered in the oncology patient. It is advantageous to wait until some healing has occurred and the ultimate position of the lips appears evident before placing implants.

PHASE III: THE AESTHETIC AND FUNCTIONAL REFINEMENT

The primary concern of this phase is usually debulking and "shaping" excess soft tissue. The first debulking procedure can be performed as early as 6 weeks following the initial flap procedure. This allows enough time roughly to gauge how much viable vascularized adipose tissue remains. If the flap has been performed for maxillary or mandibular reconstruction, the debulking often centers around vestibuloplasties in conjunction with dental rehabilitation. If osseointe-grated implants are to be placed, this is done at the time of the vestibuloplasty. Both tissue-borne dentures and osseointegrated implants require a soft tissue substrate over the bone, which is thin and immobile.[43] If a skin paddle has been used to cover bone intraorally, some form of de-bulking is frequently required. If a skin paddle has been used to cover the bony reconstruction, the subcutaneous tissue can be thinned so that the paddle overlying the denture or implant-bearing bone consists of essentially a full-thick-ness skin graft. If additional vestibular depth and satisfactory implant-bearing surface area is required, vestibuloplasties are performed. When adequate soft tissue contour is not attained with the first debulking procedure, additional debulking is performed during the second stage abutment placement when the implants are uncovered.

If a flap has been used for external soft tissue replacement, the debulking should be done very conservatively, waiting up to 6 months before the second debulking. Cutaneous skin paddles continue to loose bulk over 1 year after placement, and some skin paddle contracture also continues over this long time span. The forces of scar contracture in the severe trauma bed are extremely tenacious; what looked like adequate soft tissue contour at 3 to 6 months can become distorted at 1 year. If this is the case, it is useful to have some bulk remaining for additional surgical manipulation.

The variability in volume loss within the different vascularized soft tissues available for transfer to the head and neck is considerable. If the soft tissue component of a flap is to be used for internal volume replacement, it is crucial that vascularized adipose tissue be included either as a component of a de-epithelialized fasciocutaneous skin paddle or as subcutaneous adipose tissue transferred with a myofascial flap carrier. If the adipose tissue is transferred with muscle, the bulk of the muscle reliably decreases markedly over 6 to 8 months.[34] When the flap is being placed under native skin, the muscle should be inset lateral to the adipose tissue and skin grafted, and a tight closure to accommodate the muscle and adipose tissue should be avoided. The area that is skin grafted can be excised in several months, and the scar revised. If the vascularized adipose tissue is trimmed to obtain wound closure without skin grafting, when the muscle atrophies the volume replacement is likely deficient. The vascularized adipose tissue often not only retains its volume following transfer, but increases in volume if the patient undergoes weight gain.[44] In general, if bulk is required for contouring or filling a soft tissue

defect, the most reliable and predictable tissue to use is vascularized adipose. The final volume adjustments should always be conservative and performed no sooner than 8 to 12 months following surgery.

Unlike many oncologic ablation patients, most facial trauma patients have remaining dentition following the major reconstructive procedure. With the use of these dental abutments for reten-tion and stabilization, a trial with a tissue-borne denture is justified before subjecting the patient to the time and expense of an implant retained or implant-borne denture rehabilitation. An interim denture prosthesis can be easily fabricated for trial purposes. If it seems to function satisfactorily, a permanent tissue-borne denture is made. If not, then dental rehabilitation with implants can be started.

The major problem encountered with implant placement in the patient population with severe perioral trauma is the dynamic nature of the perio-ral healing and contracture resulting in implant placement that is too close to the final position of the lips. This problem is complicated by the neces-sary delay in final oral stoma reconstruction (so that adequate exposure to work in the oral cavity is maintained until after most of the dental rehabil-itation is done). In addition, the scarred, recon-structed oral stoma is considerably more rigid than the normal lip aperture, and nearly all patients who have had significant loss of lip and perioral soft tissue have some degree of microstomia after the final oral stoma reconstruction to prevent drooling (**Fig. 4**). If this problem is anticipated, the surgeon should place the implants on a slightly more lingual position than is normally used. Generous vestibuloplasties also help to bring the lips forward away from the implant-bearing surface of the bone.

Refinement of the nasal reconstruction is per-formed at this time (**Fig. 5**). Attaining a normal nasal structure in these patients can be extremely chal-lenging. The surrounding contracture forces distort all but the most stable underlying bone or cartilage framework. Dorsal bone grafts should be rigidly fixed to the glabellar area with miniplates of at least 1.5 mm. When cartilage grafts are used in recon-struction of the nasal ala, they should be obtained from the costal margin. Auricular and septal carti-lage are too weak to withstand the surrounding scar contracture in these sever injuries and may not maintain a satisfactory contour. If color match is poor in a transplanted skin paddle, the use of medical tattooing may be used to soften the color differences with the surrounding tissues. This should be done in a very conservative and staged fashion, initially starting in an area that is least visible.

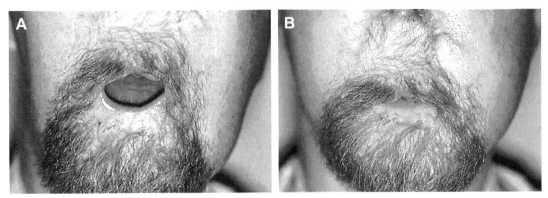

Fig. 4. (A) A 23-year-old man 14 months status postrepair of avulsive gunshot wound to mouth. Microstomia present but oral sphincter recreated. (B) Patient able to control lip function and minimize drooling and oral incompetence.

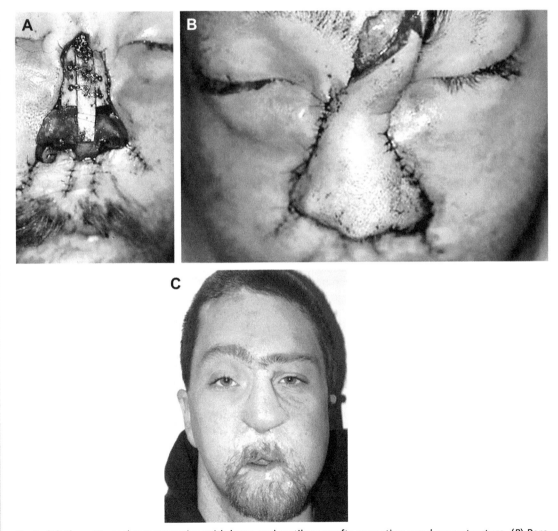

Fig. 5. (A) Phase III nasal reconstruction with bone and cartilage grafts recreating nasal suprastructure. (B) Paramedian forehead flap used for external coverage. Turbinate flaps are used for internal coverage. (C) Patient 2 years status postreconstruction.

If a facial prosthesis (for the nose or other structures) or an ocular prosthesis is to be used, these should be fabricated at this time (**Fig. 6**). The use of osseointegrated implants to anchor facial prostheses is preferred to adhesives for several reasons. The considerable forces generated by motion of facial skin tend to dislodge the facial prosthesis retained with adhesives.[45,46] Also, many patients find daily adhesive use irritating to the skin and frequently unreliable. For an ocular prosthesis to be retained and have a natural appearance, an adequate conjunctival pocket is required. When a substantial amount of the conjunctiva has been destroyed in the trauma, mucosal grafting is used to restore this depth. If possible the patient should be referred to a professional cosmetologist or counseled regarding hair style, makeup, and adjunctive measures, such as shaded glasses that enhance the positive aspects and camouflage the negative aspects of the final reconstruction.

COMPLICATIONS

The complications that may occur in the global management of severe head and neck trauma patients are extensive and beyond the scope of this article. Complications related to the reconstruction can be grouped as primarily functional or aesthetic. The functional complications may occur in the following areas: flap vascular failure, infection, vision, mastication, oral stoma competence, speech, and swallowing. The most frequent aesthetic complications encountered include poor nasal projection and shape, traumatic telecanthus, apparent asymmetry of the position of the eyes, and unsatisfactory facial contour caused by underlying bone or overlying soft tissue irregularity. Aesthetic complications, although somewhat subjective because of the nature of the patient population, should include identifiably poor aesthetic results that may have been prevented.

Factors resulting in flap failure caused by vascular complications in these cases are similar to those in oncologic reconstructions, and the principles of sound microvascular surgery should be followed. There are, however, several differences that should be mentioned. A large number of free-tissue transfer procedures following facial trauma are used to reconstruct the mid and upper face. Care should be exercised in creating a generous tunnel into the neck to ensure that the pedicle is not compressed. A tunnel entering the buccal fat pad and running out over the mandible serves this purpose. A coronoidectomy can be performed in cases of maxillary reconstruction. If any tension is anticipated on the vascular pedicle, vein grafts should be used. Following severe lower facial trauma, the submandibular triangle may be inflamed. In some cases, removal of the submandibular gland on the side of the anastomosis greatly facilitates access to branches of the external carotid (which are a safe distance from the tissues disrupted as a result of the ballistic trauma, wound contamination, and inflammation).

Infection is a constant threat in cases of severe ballistic trauma to the face. Early institution of antibiotics, debridement of nonviable tissues and foreign matter from the wound, and stabilization of fractures reduce the risk of serious infection.[12,28–30] All definitive bone grafts should be surrounded with vascularized tissue[12] and rigidly fixated. Mucosal and flap closures in the floor of the mouth must be watertight. Nonvascularized bone reconstruction of the mandible should only be undertaken in a sterile wound with satisfactory soft tissue coverage available both internally and externally. If infection does occur in the neck, prompt drainage and diversion away from the vascular pedicle should be undertaken. If the vascular pedicle is exposed to the infection, it should be covered with a pectoralis myofascial flap.

Because the tongue is usually not severely injured in most facial trauma, oral intake of nutrition and reasonable speech are usually possible once healing has occurred. The most frequent problems relating to oral function are precise

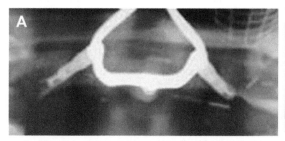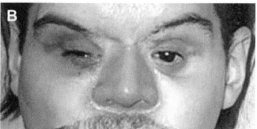

Fig. 6. (*A*) Panoramic radiograph of a patient with traumatic nasal loss with nasomaxillary osseointegrated implants and nasal suprastructure. (*B*) This patient received an osseointegrated implant-borne nasal prosthesis.

restoration of occlusion and oral stoma competence. Restoration of occlusion in remaining tooth-bearing segments depends on the early re-establishment of correct maxillomandibular relationships. Intermaxillary fixation, dental splints, and careful maintenance of centric occlusion during mandibular or maxillary reconstruction are crucial. A frequent problem in the placement of intermaxillary fixation on distal mandibular segments is excessive lingual titling of the mandibular segment when the wires are tightened. This problem can be avoided with the use of splints and careful application of intermaxillary fixation without overtightening.

Traumatic telecanthus and blunted canthal angles are among the most difficult posttraumatic deformities to correct. Establishment of a normal intercanthal distance should be done as soon as possible following injury. Revision surgery to repair traumatic telecanthus is extremely difficult, and the results are generally disappointing.

Areas of facial asymmetry resulting from atrophy of soft tissue incorporated into the reconstruction may in some cases be unpreventable. Satisfactory control of late-volume changes is possible with the appropriate selection of flap soft tissue composition. Excess volume at the initial definitive reconstruction and staged debulking over at least 6 to 12 months postoperatively should be the rule.

SUMMARY

Early aggressive surgery with immediate bone and soft tissue reconstruction is recommended for the management of extensive maxillofacial trauma (phase I). In the early period after injury, microvascular free flaps are preferred because of their excellent vascularity, good filling capacity, and the ability to transfer composite tissues specific to the defect (phase II). Patients treated with this surgical strategy develop fewer problems in the form of infection, contraction, and scarring, and require fewer secondary corrections. Successful primary treatment allows the surgeon to use multiple modalities, including tissue expansion, local flaps, and grafts, in a noninfected environment to achieve optimal function and cosmesis (phase III). The treatment is rewarding, and the results are surprisingly good when using this phased approach.

REFERENCES

1. Marciani RD. Management of midface fractures: fifty years later. J Oral Maxillofac Surg 1993;51:960–8.
2. Adams WM. Internal wiring fixation of facial fractures. Surgery 1942;12:523–40.
3. Sofferman RA, Danielson PA, Quatela V, et al. Retrospective analysis of surgically treated LeFort fractures. Arch Otolaryngol 1983;109:446–8.
4. Stanley RB Jr. Reconstruction of the midfacial vertical dimension following LeFort fractures. Arch Otolaryngol 1984;110:571–5.
5. Gruss JS, Mackinnon SE. Complex maxillary fractures: role of buttress reconstruction and immediate bone grafts. Plast Reconstr Surg 1986;78: 9–22.
6. Manson PN, Crawley WA, Yaremchuk MJ, et al. Midface fractures: advantages of immediate extended open reduction and bone grafting. Plast Reconstr Surg 1985;76:1–12.
7. Stanley RB Jr, Becker TS. Injuries of the nasofrontal orifices in frontal sinus fractures. Laryngoscope 1987;97:728–31.
8. Rahn BA. Theoretical considerations in rigid fixation of facial bones. Clin Plast Surg 1989;16:21–7.
9. Klotch DW, Gilliland R. Internal fixation vs. conventional therapy in midface fractures. J Trauma 1987; 27:1136–45.
10. Futran ND, Urken ML, Buchbinder D, et al. Rigid fixation of vascularized bone grafts in mandibular reconstruction. Arch Otolaryngol Head Neck Surg 1995;121(1):70–6.
11. Bakamjian VY, Poole M. Maxillo-facial and palatal reconstructions with the deltopectoral flap. Br J Plast Surg 1977;30(1):17–37.
12. Gruss JS, Antonyshyn O, Phillips JH. Early definitive bone and soft tissue reconstruction of major gunshot wounds of the face. Plast Reconstr Surg 1991;87: 436–50.
13. Dupoirieux L, Teot L, Jammet P, et al. The role of microsurgery in salvage operations for cranio-cerebral gunshot wounds: as case report. J Craniomaxillofac Surg 1994;22:81–5.
14. Olding M, Winski FV, Aulisi E. Emergency free flap reconstruction of a facial gunshot wound. Ann Plast Surg 1993;31:82–6.
15. Denny AD, Sanger JR, Matloub HS, et al. Self-inflicted midline facial gunshot wounds: the case for combined craniofacial and microvascular team approach. Ann Plast Surg 1992;29:564–70.
16. Vitkus K, Vitkus M. Microsurgical reconstruction of shotgun-blast wounds to the face. J Reconstr Microsurg 1990;6:279–86.
17. Urken ML. Overview of free tissue transfer. In: Urken ML, Cheney ML, Sullivan MJ, et al, editors. Atlas of regional and free flaps for head and neck reconstruction. New York: Raven Press; 1995. p. 8–35.
18. Buncke HJ. Free flap selection. In: Buncke HJ, editor. Microsurgery: transplantation-replantation. Philadelphia: Lea & Febiger; 1991. p. 102–30.
19. Thorne CH. Gunshot wounds to the face. Clin Plast Surg 1992;19(1):233–44.

20. Clark N, Birely B, Manson PN, et al. High-energy ballistic and avulsive facial injuries: classification, patterns, and an algorithm for primary reconstruction. Plast Reconstr Surg 1996;98:583–601.

21. Futran ND, Farwell DG, Smith RB, et al. Definitive management of severe facial trauma utilizing free tissue transfer. Otolaryngol Head Neck Surg 2005; 132:75–85.

22. Gaboriau HP, Kreutziger KL. Penetrating injuries of the face. J La State Med Soc 1998;150:6–9.

23. Vasconez HC, Shockley ME, Luce EA. High-energy gunshot wounds to the face. Ann Plast Surg 1996; 36:18–25.

24. Suominen E, Tukianen E. Close range shotgun and rifle injuries to the face. Clin Plast Surg 2001;28(2): 323–37.

25. Ordog FG. Penetrating neck trauma. J Trauma 1987; 27:543–54.

26. Sclafani SJA, Panetta R, Gosdstein AS, et al. The management of arterial injuries caused by penetration of zone II of the neck. J Trauma 1985;25:871–81.

27. Brackup AB, Carter KD, Nerad JA, et al. Long-term follow-up of severely injured eyes following globe rupture. Ophthal Plast Reconstr Surg 1991;7(3): 194–7.

28. Dolin J, Scalea T, Mannor L, et al. The management of gunshot wounds to the face. J Trauma 1992;33: 508–15.

29. Cole RD, Brown JF, Phipps CD. Gunshot wounds to the mandible and midface: evaluation, treatment and avoidance of complications. Otolaryngol Head Neck Surg 1994;111:739–45.

30. Kihtir T, Ivatury RR, Simon RJ, et al. Early management of civilian gunshot wounds to the face. J Trauma 1993;35:569–77.

31. Thoresby FP, Darlow HM. The mechanisms of primary infection of bullet wounds. Br J Surg 1967; 54:359–61, 32.

32. Tikka S. The contamination of missile wounds with special reference to early antimicrobial therapy. Acta Chir Scand Suppl 1982;508:281–7.

33. Daulgren B, Almskog B, Berlin R, et al. Local effects of antibacterial therapy (Benzyl-Penicillin) on missile wound infection rate and tissue devitalization when debridement is delayed for twelve hours. Acta Chir Scand Suppl 1992;508:271–9.

34. Funk FG, Laurenzo JF, Valentino J, et al. Free-tissue transfer reconstruction of midfacial and cranio-orbito-facial defects. Arch Otolaryngol Head Neck Surg 1995;121:294–303.

35. Cohen SR, Leonard DK, Markowitz BL, et al. Acrylic splints for dental alignment in complex facial injuries. Ann Plast Surg 1993;31:406–12.

36. Moscoso JF, Keller J, Genden E, et al. Vascularized bone flaps in oromandibular reconstruction. Arch Otolaryngol Head Neck Surg 1994;120:36–43.

37. Frodel JL, Funk GF, Capper DT, et al. Osseointegrated implants: a comparative study of bone thickness in four vascularized bone flaps. Plast Reconstr Surg 1993;92:449–58.

38. Roumanas ED, Nishimura R, Davis B, et al. Osseointegrated implants in the maxillary resection patient. In: Zlotlow D, editor. Proceedings of the First International Congress on Maxillofacial Prosthetics. New York: Memorial Sloan-Kettering Cancer Center; 1995. p. 36–42.

39. Futran ND, Wadsworth JT, Villaret D, et al. Midface reconstruction with the fibula free flap. Arch Otolaryngol Head Neck Surg 2002;128(2):161–6.

40. Futran ND. Retrospective case series of primary and secondary microvascular free tissue transfer reconstruction of midfacial defect. J Prosthet Dent 2001; 86(4):369–76.

41. Goodrich JT, Argamaso R, Hall CD. Split thickness bone grafts in complex craniofacial reconstructions. Pediatr Neurosurg 1992;18:195–201.

42. Szachowicz EH. Facial bone wound healing. Otolaryngol Clin North Am 1995;28:865–80.

43. Urken ML, Buchbinder D, Weinberg H, et al. Primary placement of osseointegrated implants in microvascular mandibular reconstruction. Otolaryngol Head Neck Surg 1989;101:56–73.

44. Mordick TG II, Larossa D, Whitaker L. Soft-tissue reconstruction of the face: a comparison of dermal-fat grafting and vascularized tissue transfer. Ann Plast Surg 1992;29:390–6.

45. Jensen TO, Brown C, Blacker J. Nasofacial prostheses supported by osseointegrated implants. Int J Oral Maxillofac Implants 1992;7:203–11.

46. Moy PK, Lundgren S, Beumer J, et al. Stabilization of craniofacial prostheses using osseointegrated titanium implants. Laryngoscope 1993;103:1399–405.

Reconstruction of Periauricular and Temporal Bone Defects

Tim A. Iseli, MBBS, FRACS, Eben L. Rosenthal, MD*

KEYWORDS

- Reconstruction • Free flap • Periauricular
- Temporal bone • Cutaneous malignancy • Ear • Parotid

CLASSIFICATION OF THE DEFECT

The internal skull base is divided anatomically into three fossa: anterior, middle, and posterior. From a surgical perspective, the skull base also may be divided into three regions based on the growth pattern of malignancies (**Fig. 1**). Region I comprises the orbital roof and cribiform plate and typically is involved by sinonasal tumors. Region II commonly is involved by infratemporal fossa tumors extending superiorly. Region III includes the temporal bone with extension into posterior and middle cranial fossa. This region typically is involved by tumors invading the external auditory canal or temporal bone. For the purposes of this discussion, the lateral skull base is defined as regions II and III.

Although there are a variety of tumor types that affect the lateral skull base in adults, the most common are squamous cell carcinoma, followed by basal cell carcinoma, and then various parotid malignancies extending into the deep tissue.[1] In the pediatric population, skin cancers are rare with lymphomas, sarcomas, neuroblastomas, and nasopharyngeal tumors more common; many of these are treated primarily nonsurgically (with the exception of biopsy and refractory cases).

A defect classification system has been proposed to predict the preferred reconstructive technique based on the size and volume of resection. Defects may be classified as class I: preauricular with preservation of the external auditory canal; class II: lateral temporal bone resection with middle ear obliteration and preservation of much of the pinna; and class III: total auriculectomy with significant volume loss from parotidectomy, temporal bone resection with or without temporomandibular joint, and zygoma resection. Reconstruction aims to cover the cutaneous defect and adjacent vital structures with the ability to heal in an irradiated field and withstand further treatment if required.

CONSIDERATIONS DURING RESECTION

Recurrent or advanced stage primary cutaneous lesions or periparotid metastatic squamous cell carcinoma tumors often demand large resections involving skin, parotid tissue, or masseter and often underlying bone, including the ramus of the mandible and portions of the temporal bone. Resecting surgeons may improve the final reconstructive result significantly by sparing part or all of the facial nerve (if functional preoperatively) and, where possible, a small strip of the superior part of the pinna (for support of glasses).

Preservation of the external ear canal and tympanic membrane (with attached malleous and incus) are less important as the resultant conductive hearing loss is generally well restored with amplification. Patients having difficulty with monaural hearing may benefit from a cross aid or a bone conduction, or bone-anchored, hearing aid (BAHA). A quality-of-life analysis showed that patients who had preserved sensorineural hearing benefitted significantly from a BAHA, which may be placed at the time of resection.[2] The BAHA peg ideally should be applied outside the radiation

Division of Otolaryngology, Head & Neck Surgery, Department of Surgery, University of Alabama School of Medicine, BDB 563, 1530 3rd Avenue South, Birmingham, AL 35294-0012, USA
* Corresponding author.
E-mail address: eben.rosenthal@ccc.uab.edu (E.L. Rosenthal).

Facial Plast Surg Clin N Am 17 (2009) 253–262
doi:10.1016/j.fsc.2009.01.005

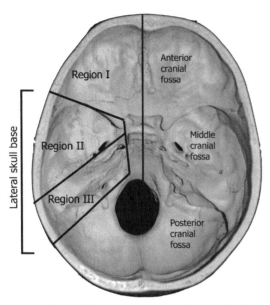

Fig. 1. Division of the anterior and middle cranial fossa into three regions based on the common growth patterns of malignancies. The lateral skull base is defined as regions II and III.

field; otherwise, the inset tends to work loose over a period of years as a result of vibration of the aid.

Functional outcomes after resection of the mandibular condyle and posterior ramus usually are satisfactory without anatomic reconstruction. In patients who have teeth, maxillomandibular fixation for 2 to 6 weeks may prevent malocclusion resulting from the pull of pterygoid muscles but this must be weighed against the risks for worsening trismus in irradiated patients.[3]

RECONSTRUCTIVE OPTIONS

The goals of reconstruction for lateral temporal bone defects are well understood (**Box 1**). Although bone commonly is removed during ablation, the focus of lateral temporal bone reconstructions is on replacement of skin and soft tissue. Significant deep soft tissue resections with minimal skin loss should be reconstructed with soft tissue alone to improve healing and cosmetic outcomes by introducing vascularized tissue and obliterating dead space. Careful defect analysis is required before deciding on the best reconstructive option (**Box 2**). Because the majority of patients who have periauricular and temporal bone defects are elderly, the goal of reconstruction is to facilitate rapid, reliable healing and functional outcomes rather than cosmesis. Reconstructive options include primary closure, skin grafting, local flaps, regional flaps, and free tissue transfer (**Box 3**).

Box 1
Goals of reconstruction

Bring vascularized tissue into a heavily irradiated field

Withstand further radiotherapy

Cover large cutaneous defect with satisfactory contour and cosmesis

Separate the aerodigestive tract

Cover dura and prevent cerebrospinal fluid (CSF) leaks

Cover carotid artery

Support glasses and prosthetics

Compensate for loss of facial nerve function

Preserve or allow for future restoration of hearing when possible

PRIMARY CLOSURE AND SKIN GRAFTING

Primary closures may be achieved with preauricular defects using wide undermining of the face deep to the superficial musculoaponeurotic system (SMAS). Plication of the SMAS layer prevents excess tension on the skin edges. A tension-free repair is especially important in irradiated tissue because of higher wound complications.

The scalp offers less laxity for primary closure. Galeal-releasing incisions performed parallel to the incised edge at 1-cm intervals allow some reach while preserving adequate blood supply to the wound edge. Tissue expanders provide additional reach for primary closure but may delay wound healing and thereby delay radiotherapy start.[4]

Box 2
Defect analysis in lateral temporal bone reconstruction

Dural resection or CSF leak

Facial nerve transection

Size and location of skin loss

Soft tissue loss

Mandibular ramus

External auditory canal presence

Middle ear ablation

Partial loss of the auricle

Other cranial nerve deficits

Box 3
Reconstructive options for lateral skull base defects

Primary closure

Skin grafts

Local and regional flaps

    Temporalis muscle flap

    Pectoralis myofacial or myocutaneous flap

    Cervicofacial rotation flap

    Keystone design perforator island flap

    Latissimus dorsi myofacial flap

    Trapezius cutaneous flap

    Sternomastoid myofacial flap

    Galeal superficial temporal artery flap

Free tissue transfer

    Rectus flap

    Anterior lateral thigh flap

    Radial forearm free flap

Skin graft survival is variable directly onto cranial bone and may be improved by rotating in pedicled pericranium or by burring down the calvarium to bleeding marrow. Komorowska-Timek and colleagues[5] described complete survival of all split-thickness skin grafts in four nonirradiated full-thickness scalp defects using artifical dermis. A delay to skin grafting, however, often was required and the split-thickness skin graft may not withstand postoperative radiotherapy or have the bulk to replace larger volume defects.[6]

As patients who have cutaneous malignancy have a high rate of synchronous or metachronous tumors, skin grafting and primary closure have the advantage of preserving future reconstructive options, facilitating monitoring for recurrence, and shortening operative time for patients who have significant medical comorbidities. Partial wound breakdown, skin graft failure, or general poor wound healing can be managed effectively using negative pressure dressings.[7] Split-thickness skin graft survival can be improved with the use of negative pressure dressings.[8,9]

LOCAL AND REGIONAL FLAPS

Local and regional flaps are a good alternative to free flap reconstruction, especially for elderly patients for whom a short operative time is desirous or where vascular disease may compromise arterial patency. They require incision planning in conjunction with a resecting surgeon and generally provide excellent color match for smaller-volume defects with lower distant morbidity. The well-vascularized nature of the scalp and cervical skin allows longer random pattern paddles with smaller pedicles than would survive elsewhere in the body. Again, galeal-releasing incisions made 1 cm apart can be used to increase the rotational arch or ability of local flaps to close scalp defects.

The temporalis muscle flap is a good option for soft tissue around the temporal bone and has been used to line intraoral defects; however, this flap has a limited reach, little final bulk, and results in a cosmetic temporal "hollowing" that may be partly camouflaged by hair styling.[10] The temporalis muscle transposition also is used to fill exenterated orbits or as part of dynamic facial reanimation.

The sternomastoid flap has limited bulk and caudal reach, especially after neck dissection. The lower trapezius myocutaneous island flap is pedicled on the descending branch of the transverse cervical artery and has similarly limited bulk, arc, and viability in the previously operated neck.[11] Platysmal fasciocutaneous flaps, such as the inferiorly based occipital rotation flap, often require split skin grafting to the donor site, which may break down if inside the radiation field.[12] The galeal superficial temporal artery flap is a thin flap that relies on a blood supply that may be compromised during the resection and provides little bulk.[13]

The keystone design perforator island flap is a versatile islanded skin and SMAS flap that may be undermined to 50% of its length to allow rotation. Its donor site generally is closed primarily with a double-ended V to Y closure.[14] This requires the skin laxity often present in elderly patients who have periauricular cutanous malignancies but may be limited by previous tumors or other surgeries in the region.

Perhaps the most commonly used local flap in the authors' institution is the cervicofacial rotation flap. It can cover large defects and is robust and reliable within a heavily irradiated field.[15] Extension of the incision onto the chest improves reach and vascularity of this flap.

Box 4
Indications for free tissue transfer

Previously heavily irradiated or operated field

Planned postoperative radiation therapy

Large soft tissue or cutaneous deficit

Vital underlying structures (eg, exposed carotid or dura)

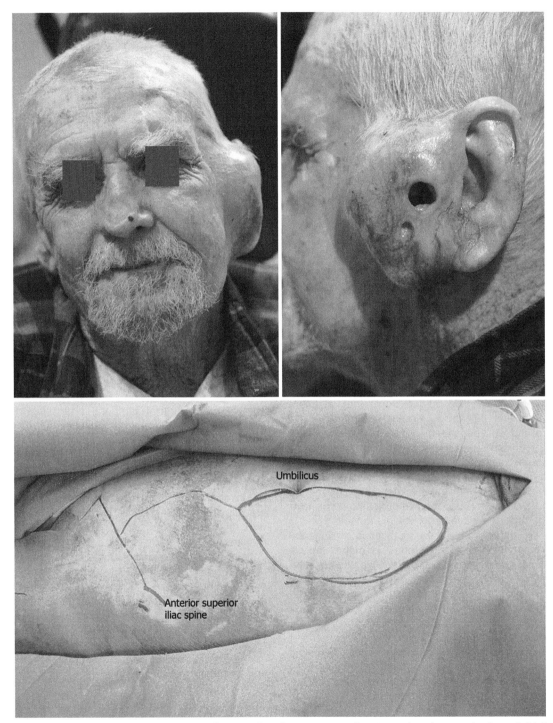

Fig. 2. Lateral temporal bone resection with rectus free flap reconstruction. Note that the anterior lateral thigh also can be prepped out with the rectus flap if there is uncertainty about the size of the defect.

A cervicofacial rotational flap can be used to reconstruct most skin-only defects in this region, but the reliability may be reduced by previous radiation treatment or smoking. If the facial artery is sacrificed during neck dissection, the vascularity of the flap may be reduced further and the risk for partial flap loss increased.

Although the soft tissue component of the wound often is not well addressed by cervicofacial rotation flap alone, pectoralis major myofascial

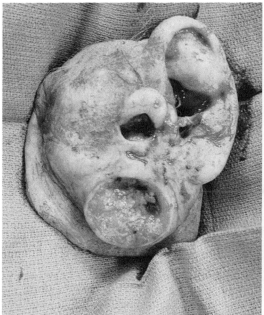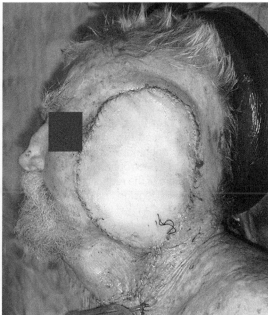

Fig. 2. (*continued*)

flap may be used concurrently for bulk.[16] The pectoralis major flap is extremely reliable as a myofascial flap in combination with skin grafting or as a myocutaneous flap for soft tissue bulk. Both flaps have caudal limitation, with reduced survival and increased dehiscence above the lower edge of the zygoma. A staged procedure may allow use of the pectoralis myofacial flap above the temporal line.[17]

MICROVASCULAR FREE TISSUE TRANSFER

Free flap reconstruction should be considered when defects are large, postoperative radiation therapy is anticipated, or the area has been previously radiated (**Box 4**). Overall, free flaps have become the gold standard for repair of larger periauricular defects. There have been improvements in the speed and cost of free flap reconstruction since their inception in the late 1960's.[18] It provides the greatest flexibility in size, bulk, and reach with high reliability even in elderly patients.[19] Free flaps bring vascularized tissue into previously irradiated fields and may allow reirradiation with less wound morbidity. There usually are recipient arterial vessels readily available from the external carotid system and draining veins into the internal or external jugular network. The classification system described above has been used to determine the type of free flap reconstruction used.[20]

The radial forearm free flap provides extremely robust, thin skin ideal for a class I defect. It has a long vascular pedicle and may be harvested simultaneously with low donor-site morbidity.[21] Its pedicle may be divided 2 weeks after inset (unlike the rectus abdominis flap) and the skin may be perforated or folded (unlike the anterolateral thigh) to allow reconstruction of part of the external auditory canal. The lateral arm free flap offers comparatively increased volume and the possibility of sensory reinnervation but with less size than the anterolateral thigh.[22] Because its vessels are small and its pedicle length short, it largely has been replaced by the anterolateral thigh at our institution.

The anterior lateral thigh probably is the ideal reconstructive flap for medium-sized defects with significant cutaneous involvement (class II). This flap has moderate soft tissue volume and allows for a long skin paddle although width is limited to 8 to 10 cm to allow for primary closure of the donor site. If the soft tissue defect is large and no skin reconstruction is required, this flap can be de-epithelized and a small skin paddle left externally for monitoring purposes. Implantable Doppler probes also are appropriate for flaps that are buried or have limited visibility for monitoring. The anterior lateral thigh flap can be harvested simultaneously and offers reduced donor-site morbidity compared with the radial forearm free flap because the donor site can be closed primarily.[23]

Thickness of the anterolateral thigh flap varies significantly with gender and body habitus, which makes the flap extremely thick in obese women.

The rectus abdominis free flap allows for simultaneous harvest of a very large volume with a large skin paddle for class III defects (**Fig. 2**).[24] Rectus abdominis free flaps often require secondary debulking as the muscular atrophy is variable. The donor site leaves a large incision and tight closure of the abdomen may lead to pain and increased risk for atelectasis, pneumonia, and later hernia formation.[25] This has led to routine use of polypropylene mesh in closure of the rectus sheath layer in an attempt to reduce tension, pain, and subsequent hernia formation.

CONSIDERATIONS IN FLAP RECONSTRUCTION
General Considerations

Class I, mostly cutaneous defects involving the cheek or superficial parotid, can be reconstructed with a cervicofacial flap, a radial forearm free flap, or the anterior lateral thigh flap. Any dead space should be obliterated carefully by deep sutures securing the flap facia against strong underlying tissues (eg, facia or periosteum). Secure sutures on the cranial aspect prevent the effects of gravity over time on larger grafts or those pedicled inferiorly. Securing the deep fascia on the flap to periosteum of the zygoma or orbital floor helps prevents lower eyelid ectropion for the same reason.

The radial forearm flap has the advantage of a large surface area of thin tissue. Larger volume defects are best reconstructed using anterior lateral thigh or rectus flaps depending on a patient's body habitus. These flaps tend to be bulky but it is better to overfill than underfill these defects as most shrink after muscular denervation atrophy and radiotherapy. Secondary debulking procedures to obtain appropriate facial contour are easily performed on an outpatient basis under local anesthesia and are well tolerated. In the authors' institution, approximately 30% of patients undergoing rectus abdominis free flaps require a revision procedure.

Dural Defects

Bony reconstruction of the temporoparietal calvarium when there is dural exposure remains controversial and not used frequently in the authors' practice. Synthetic materials, acellular bone matrices, or titanium mesh have been used to cover the dura and protect the underlying brain. Unfortunately, all these materials have shown a high propensity to become exposed and subsequently infected in irradiated fields.[26] Titanium mesh limits the usefulness of postoperative CT scans, which often are useful for tumor surveillance, especially in delineating bony anatomy. Titanium mesh has less effect on MRI scanning but MRI has less usefulness in imaging bone.

Dural openings within the defect often require a separate fascial repair in combination with free tissue transfer. Pericranium is vascularized and robust; however, synthetic materials, allograft, and xenograft material remain widely used. Alternatively, fascia can be harvested from the rectus site or from the anterior lateral thigh donor site and used as a patch repair with the free flap tissue then placed over the repair. The flap should be secured to surrounding bone by passing sutures through holes drilled in the outer table to prevent dead space in which CSF might collect.

Facial Nerve Considerations

Extensive lateral skull base resections often result in temporary or permanent facial nerve weakness. A lengthy discussion of facial nerve reanimation is beyond the scope of this article but a brief discussion of commonly used concurrent ancillary procedures is warranted.

When a segment of the facial nerve is resected with the specimen, immediate primary anastomosis or interposition grafting provides the best results even if the region has been previously irradiated as the distal nerves are easiest to identify and stimulate. The greater auricular nerve may lie too close to a tumor to be oncologically safe and a nerve near the free tissue harvest site often is available and prevents the additional morbidity of a second donor site (**Table 1**). Unfortunately, patients have to wait 12 to 18 months before return of function and results are significantly worse in patients over age 60, who represent the majority of patients who have advanced periauricular cutaneous malignancies.[27]

If facial nerve interposition is not possible because of absence of the proximal nerve, early anastamosis from part of the hypoglossal to the distal stump should be considered in young patients who have a reasonable prognosis. Secondary procedures also can be considered in patients who have a good prognosis, including a cross-facial nerve graft or free muscle transfer.

Ancillary Procedures

Several ancillary procedures should be considered when the facial nerve cannot be repaired or when a delayed return of function is expected. Functional recovery of facial nerve grafting often depends on age and pre- or postoperative radiation therapy. Patients over age 60 who have poor prognoses are offered immediate static

Table 1	
Facial nerve graft options	
Radial Forearm Free Flap	**Medial and Brachial Cutaneous Nerve**
Anterior lateral thigh flap	Nerve to vastus lateralis
Rectus muscle	Nerve to rectus muscle *or* separate nerve graft site
Local flap	Greater auricular nerve Distant nerve graft site (eg, sural nerve)

reanimation with lateral canthopexy and gold weight placement for ocular protection. If not performed at the time of surgery, canthopexy and gold weight implantation should be performed within several weeks of the initial surgery to prevent corneal exposure keratitis. Patients who have associated fifth nerve anesthesia are at even higher risk for corneal damage and should be treated proactively. Every patient should be discharged with eye care instructions, including lubricant and routine precautions against corneal exposure.

A midface sling using heavy prolene sutures from the dermis of the nasolabial fold vertically to the periosteum of the orital floor improves cosmesis and aids oral competence. The sutures should exceed the desired oral commissure elevation as there tends to be relaxation in the following weeks. A static sling of the lateral nasal valve often improves nasal breathing significantly. This may be performed in conjunction with a facial sling or as a separate procedure.

Auricular reconstruction often is limited by the lack of underlying bone for osteointegrated implantation or contraindicated by previous radiation. For patients concerned about cosmesis, a multistep bone-anchored prosthetic ear provides the best appearance. Otherwise, in this age group, a prosthesis may be suspended from glasses if the top part of the pinna is preserved. Less success has been observed using a tissue adhesive.

External Auditory Canal

If the tympanic membrane is left intact but the cartilaginous portion of the external auditory canal has been resected, continuity of the canal must be re-established. This can be performed by perforation of the flap and development of skin flaps for external auditory meatoplasty. The radial forearm flap or cervical facial rotation flap can be perforated but others cannot. Often, split-thickness skin grafting is required when the rectus or anterior lateral thigh flap is used.

Postoperative stenosis is common with these repairs and often requires revisions. External packing of the external auditory canal using nasal packing is important in the immediate postoperative period. The best preventative of restenosis is wide meatoplasty but creating a large perforation within the flap tissue risks devascularizing the flap.

Middle ear exposure as part of resection requires obliteration of the middle ear space and closure of the eustachian tube by scarifying the mucosa and placing a muscle plug within the lumen. If part of the pinna remains, it should be placed over de-epithelized portions of the flap to optimize contour.

Postoperative Care

Use of free flap reconstructions in temporal bone defects differs from that in patients who have upper aerodigestive tract head and neck reconstructions. There is less risk for salivary contamination and, therefore, infection. A 4- to 5-day hospital stay usually is appropriate. It is critical for patients to ambulate on postoperative day 1 to prevent venous thrombosis or chest complications and begin advancing diet as tolerated (although a soft diet for 6 weeks is recommended for comfort if the temporomandibular joint is compromised). Cranial nerve deficits associated with skull base resection or intraoperative retraction may result in aspiration and dysphagia. In these cases, a swallowing evaluation early in the hospitalization is important to determine if placement of nasal gastric feeding tube or a percutaneous endoscopic gastronomy tube is required.

Complications

Complications occur in 11% to 68% of lateral skull base surgeries. Wound healing complications are most common (**Box 5**); typical complications include partial or complete flap failure and ear canal stenosis or recurrent otitis externa. Late

Box 5
Wound healing considerations
Recurrent or future adjacent tumors
Prior radiation therapy
Planned postoperative radiation therapy
Previous surgical excisions
Medical comorbidities (hypothyroidism or malnutrition)

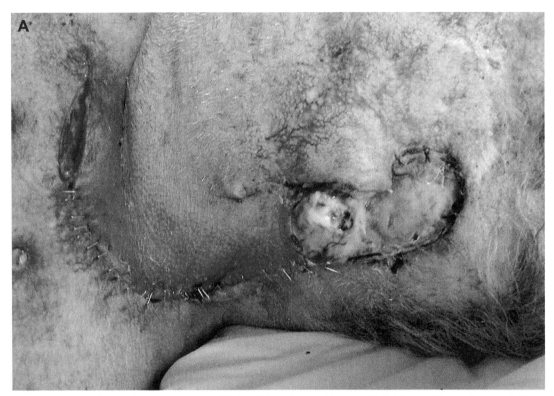

Fig. 3. Wound healing problems can occur with local flap closure. Here a split-thickness skin graft and rotational flap was used for reconstruction and the flap failed to heal onto the underlying irradiated tissue. Negative pressure dressings were used to manage this problem rather than additional surgical procedures. (*A*) Wound breakdown and nonhealing areas with slough overlying in the irradiated field (*B*) Negative-pressure dressing in-situ (*C*) Cut out of sponge used in dressing (*D*) Slough has been removed after 1 week of negative-pressure dressing allowing for a healing base to be seen.

complications may be related to the loss of facial nerve function (eg, ectropion) or related to the donor site (eg, abdominal hernia or skin graft loss). The patients treated at the authors' institution typically have had prior radiotherapy (12%) or surgery and radiation therapy (29%). Overall, approximately 5% of patients had wound healing problems that required intervention, most often related to tumor recurrence. Wound healing problems often are managed best initially with negative pressure dressings (**Fig. 3**).[7,28]

Bone exposure can be related to osteoradionecrosis or recurrent disease. If recurrent disease has been eliminated as a source of poor wound healing, hyperbaric oxygen therapy can be considered. There is concern, however, that it may promote tumor recurrence if the tumor has recently been resected.

The anterolateral thigh flap provides the best donor-site morbidity as most can be closed primarily. The radial forearm donor site is conspicuous and may be irritated by a shirt cuff. Most donor-site morbidity responds to local

wound care. Partial or total flap loss occurs in less than 5% of free flaps and may be salvaged with a pectoralis myocutaneous flap or with conservative wound management. As discussed previously, the authors have found vacuum-assisted dressings particularly useful in treating such wound problems. Secondary procedures and debulking are required most commonly in rectus abominis flaps (32%) because of their bulk and variable muscle atrophy and less commonly in anterolateral thigh flaps (13%), especially in obese patients.

Ear canal stenosis and chronic otitis externa or temporal bone osteoradionecrosis after high radiation doses remain challenging problems. In elderly patients who have satisfactory hearing in the contralateral ear, these problems are avoided by obliteration of the external canal. Many of those who have problematic external auditory canal skin respond to local treatment (cleaning, keeping the ear dry, and topical antibiotics/antiseptics) with delayed obliteration reserved for refractory cases.

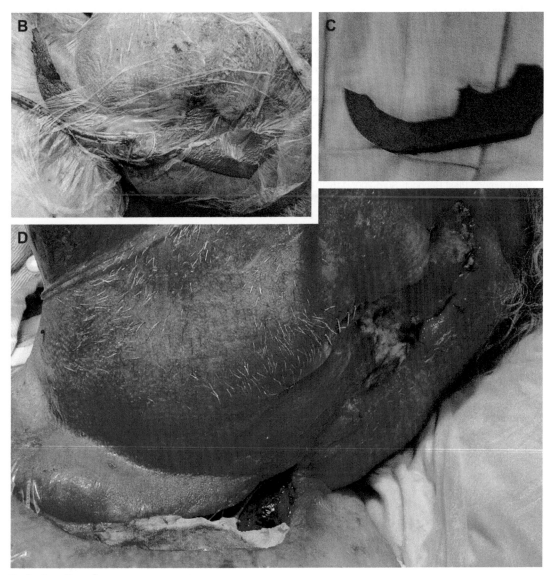

Fig. 3. (*continued*)

SUMMARY

Large periauricular and temporal bone defects most commonly follow resection of advanced non-melanoma skin cancers. Defects may be classified as class I: preauricular with preservation of the external auditory canal; class II: lateral temporal bone resection with middle ear obliteration and preservation of much of the pinna; and class III: total auriculectomy with significant volume loss from parotidectomy, temporal bone resection with or without temporomandibular joint, and zygoma resection. Reconstruction aims to cover the cutaneous defect and adjacent vital structures with the ability to heal in an irradiated field and withstand further treatment if required. The authors' preferred reconstructions are class I, cervicofacial rotation or radial forearm free flap; class II, antero-lateral thigh; and class III, rectus abominis free flap. Ancillary procedures, especially for associated facial paralysis, often are required. Although free flap reconstruction provides rapid wound healing, local and regional flaps are alternatives for patients unable to tolerate prolonged anesthesia and for use after recurrence or complications.

REFERENCES

1. Moore MG, Deschler DG, McKenna MJ, et al. Management outcomes following lateral temporal bone resection for ear and temporal bone malignancies. Otolaryngol Head Neck Surg 2007;137:893–8.

2. McLarnon CM, Davison T, Johnson IJ. Bone-anchored hearing aid: comparison of benefit by patient subgroups. Laryngoscope 2004;114:942–4.

3. Imazawa T, Komuro Y, Inoue M, et al. Mandibular fractures treated with maxillomandibular fixation screws (MMFS method). J Craniofac Surg 2006;17:544–9.

4. Chiang YC. Combined tissue expansion and prelamination of forearm flap in major ear reconstruction. [see comment]. Plast Reconstr Surg 2006;117:1292–5.

5. Komorowska-Timek E, Gabriel A, Bennett DC, et al. Artificial dermis as an alternative for coverage of complex scalp defects following excision of malignant tumors. Plast Reconstr Surg 2005;115:1010–7.

6. Rudolph R. Complications of surgery for radiotherapy skin damage. Plast Reconstr Surg 1982;70:179–85.

7. Rosenthal EL, Blackwell KE, McGrew B, et al. Use of negative pressure dressings in head and neck reconstruction. Head Neck 2005;27:970–5.

8. Andrews BT, Smith RB, Chang KE, et al. Management of the radial forearm free flap donor site with the vacuum-assisted closure (VAC) system. Laryngoscope 2006;116:1918.

9. Vidrine DM, Kaler S, Rosenthal EL. A comparison of negative-pressure dressings versus Bolster and splinting of the radial forearm donor site. Otolaryngol Head Neck Surg 2005;133:403–6.

10. Abubaker AO, Abouzgia MB. The temporalis muscle flap in reconstruction of intraoral defects: an appraisal of the technique. Oral Surg Oral Med Oral Pathol Oral Radiol Endod 2002;94:24–103.

11. Cummings CW, Eisele DW, Coltrera MD. Lower trapezius myocutaneous island flap. Arch Otolaryngol Head Neck Surg 1989;115:1181–5.

12. Moore MG, Lin DT, Mikulec AA, et al. The occipital flap for reconstruction after lateral temporal bone resection. Arch Otolaryngol Head Neck Surg 2008;134: 587–91.

13. Nayak VK, Deschler DG. Pedicled temporoparietal fascial flap reconstruction of select intraoral defects. Laryngoscope 2004;114:1545–8.

14. Pelissier P, Gardet H, Pinsolle V, et al. The keystone design perforator island flap. Part II: clinical applications. J Plast Reconstr Aesthet Surg 2007;60:888–91.

15. Moore BA, Wine T, Netterville JL. Cervicofacial and cervicothoracic rotation flaps in head and neck reconstruction. Head Neck 2005;27:1092–101.

16. Liu R, Gullane P, Brown D, et al. Pectoralis major myocutaneous pedicled flap in head and neck reconstruction: retrospective review of indications and results in 244 consecutive cases at the Toronto General Hospital. J Otolaryngol 2001;30:34–40.

17. Resto VA, McKenna MJ, Deschler DG. Pectoralis major flap in composite lateral skull base defect reconstruction. Arch Otolaryngol Head Neck Surg 2007;133:490–4.

18. Rosenthal E, Carroll W, Dobbs M, et al. Simplifying head and neck microvascular reconstruction. Head Neck 2004;26:930–6.

19. Ozkan O, Ozgentas HE, Islamoglu K, et al. Experiences with microsurgical tissue transfers in elderly patients. Microsurgery 2005;25:390–5.

20. Rosenthal EL, King T, McGrew BM, et al. Evolution of a paradigm for free tissue transfer reconstruction of lateral temporal bone defects. Head Neck 2008; 30:589–94.

21. Moscoso JF, Urken ML. Radial forearm flaps. Otolaryngol Clin North Am 1994;27:1119–40.

22. Marques Faria JC, Rodrigues ML, Scopel GP, et al. The versatility of the free lateral arm flap in head and neck soft tissue reconstruction: clinical experience of 210 cases. J Plast Reconstr Aesthet Surg 2008;61:172–9.

23. Lueg EA. The anterolateral thigh flap: radial forearm's "big brother" for extensive soft tissue head and neck defects. Arch Otolaryngol Head Neck Surg 2004;130:813–8.

24. Kroll SS, Baldwin BJ. Head and neck reconstruction with the rectus abdominis free flap. Clin Plast Surg 1994;21:97–105.

25. Wax MK, Burkey BB, Bascom D, et al. The role of free tissue transfer in the reconstruction of massive neglected skin cancers of the head and neck. Arch Facial Plast Surg 2003;5:479–82.

26. Kontio R. Treatment of orbital fractures: the case for reconstruction with autogenous bone. J Oral Maxillofac Surg 2004;62:863–8.

27. Gagnon NB, Molina-Negro P. Facial reinnervation after facial paralysis: is it ever too late? Arch Otorhinolaryngol 1989;246:303–7.

28. Shreenivas S, Magnuson JS, Rosenthal EL. Use of negative-pressure dressings to manage a difficult surgical neck wound. Ear Nose Throat J 2006;85: 390–1.

Parotid Defects

Tamer Ghanem, MD

KEYWORDS

- Parotid defects • Parotidectomy
- Cheek skin resection • Facial nerve

Two reconstructive issues must be considered following a superficial parotidectomy—prevention of Frey's syndrome and maintenance of facial contour. The earliest description of Frey's syndrome was in 1757 by Duphenix. This syndrome, also known as gustatory sweating, is named after the Polish neurologist Lucja Frey who first associated the parasympathetic fibers carried by the auriculotemporal nerve to the parotid with this syndrome in 1923. Patients notice perspiration and flushing on the affected cheek during meals. The mechanism of Frey's syndrome is believed to be aberrant reinnervation of severed postganglionic parasympathetic nerve fibers to sympathetic nerve terminals on sweat glands of elevated cheek skin. The average incidence based on subjective patient reports is 38%. When objective testing is performed, the incidence is much higher at 86%.[1,2]

The post parotidectomy sunken cheek appearance can be distressing to esthetically demanding patients undergoing surgery for benign disease, as demonstrated in **Fig. 1**. This appearance depends on the volume of parotid tissue and tumor resected. For small tail-of-parotid resections, this might not be an issue; however, in a total parotidectomy defect, surgery can leave the patient with a large asymmetric facial contour.

Various surgical approaches have been studied to decrease the incidence of Frey's syndrome and improve postoperative cosmesis. These approaches generally involve placing an allogeneic or autogenic barrier between the remaining parotid tissue and the skin flap. The most common allogeneic barrier is AlloDerm (LifeCell Corporation, The Woodlands, Texas), which is a human-derived acellular dermal tissue substitute. The advantage of this method of reconstruction is that it does not involve donor site morbidity and adds minimal time to the procedure. It is limited by its small volume, the potential for infection, and resorption over time. Govindaraj[2] prospectively studied two groups (n = 32 in each) undergoing superficial parotidectomy. One group was reconstructed with AlloDerm at the time of the ablative procedure, and a control group was not reconstructed. There was a reduction of subjective Frey's syndrome from 9% in the control group to 3% in the AlloDerm group. The objective incidence was 40% in the control group, whereas the AlloDerm group had a 0% incidence of Frey's syndrome. There was a significantly higher incidence of seromas in the AlloDerm group when compared with the control group (25% versus 9%).

Autogenic substances include abdominal fat grafts and sternocleidomastoid muscle (SCM) flaps. Studies of abdominal fat grafts have been associated with mixed reviews. Most commonly, fat is harvested from the abdomen through a small periumbilical incision (**Fig. 2**). Generally, 15% to 25% excess volume of fat is harvested to allow for a symmetrical appearance after wound healing and fat resorption. Curry and colleagues[3] studied fat graft reconstruction after superficial parotidectomy and reported decreased symptomatic Frey's syndrome in the fat graft group when compared with controls (6.3% versus 18.6%); however, this difference did not reach statistical significance. A telephone survey questionnaire of facial symmetry revealed less facial asymmetry in the fat graft group versus the controls (9% versus 39%, $P = 0.002$). The disadvantages of the abdominal fat graft are the requirement of a second incision with potential donor morbidity of a second scar, abdominal contour irregularity, and the potential for infection or hematoma.

The SCM flap has been described in reconstructing the parotid defect to aid in facial contour symmetry and to decrease the incidence of Frey's syndrome. Jost and colleagues[4] were the first to

Department of Otolaryngology-Head and Neck Surgery, Oregon Health & Science University, Portland, OR, USA
E-mail address: TGhanem1@hfhs.org

Facial Plast Surg Clin N Am 17 (2009) 263–269
doi:10.1016/j.fsc.2009.01.004
1064-7406/09/$ – see front matter © 2009 Published by Elsevier Inc.

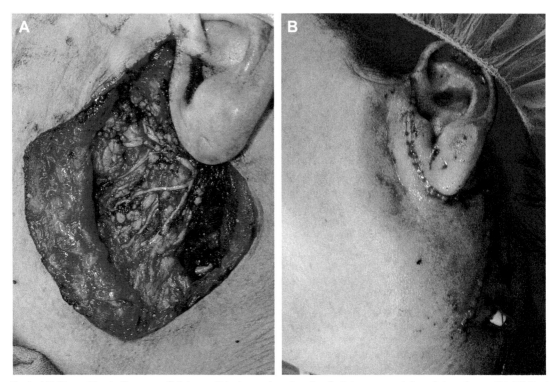

Fig. 1. (A) Wound bed after superficial parotidectomy showing the facial nerve and deep lobe of parotid. (B) Post superficial parotidectomy facial contour asymmetry or "divot" appearance.

describe a superiorly based SCM flap for reconstructing the post parotidectomy wound bed. Casler and Conley studied the SCM flap versus superficial musculoaponeurotic system (SMAS) placation, with 16 patients in each group, and compared these techniques with historical controls.[5] The incidence of Frey's syndrome was 47.1% in the control group, 12.5% in the SCM flap group, and 0% in the SMAS plication group. There was no statistical difference between the SCM flap group and the SMAS plication group. The SCM flap technique can be performed with a superiorly or inferiorly based pedicle. The superiorly based SCM flap is demonstrated in **Fig. 3**. Care must be taken to avoid injury to the spinal accessory nerve. The flap is rotated and advanced to fill the defect and sutured to the remaining SMAS layer and ear cartilage. The advantage of this technique over the abdominal fat graft is the avoidance of a second incision and its associated comorbidities. Disadvantages include the risk of spinal accessory nerve injury, the atrophy and resorption of a portion of the muscle flap, and the extent of neck dissection to free the SCM muscle.

The SMAS plication technique is limited to small posteriorly based parotid lesions. This technique requires elevating preauricular skin in a subcutaneous plane, followed by elevating the SMAS as a separate layer off the parotidomassetric fascia. It is essential to ensure that tumor does not involve the SMAS layer when performing this type of reconstruction. Once the tumor is excised, the elevated SMAS layer is plicated onto itself and the mastoid periosteum and fascia over the SCM tendon. This maneuver masks the area of the defect and maintains contour. The advantage of this technique is that it does not require a second incision or additional neck dissection. The

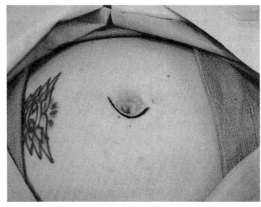

Fig. 2. A periumbilical incision is made for harvest of an abdominal fat graft.

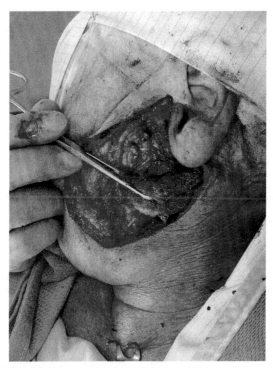

Fig. 3. A superiorly based left SCM flap is brought up to the parotid bed.

main limitation is that it is only good for small parotid defects. Also, the tumor margins must not be contiguous with the SMAS layer.

Another option for reconstructing the post superficial parotidectomy defect is a deepithelialized radial forearm free flap. The flap is harvested based on the radial artery and vena comitans in the usual manner. The flap can be anastamosed to the superficial temporal vessels or the facial vessel by the body of the mandible. A No. 10 blade is used to deepithelialize the flap, allowing the surgeon to contour the flap to the tissue defect. Multiple tacking sutures are used to tack the flap to the SMAS or remaining parotidomasseteric fascia. The main advantage of this reconstructive method is the ability to precisely fill the volume defect without having to worry about tissue shrinkage effects exhibited by the fat graft and SCM flaps. The disadvantages include a longer hospital stay for flap monitoring and donor site morbidity. This option is controversial due to the disadvantages listed, but it has been performed in a handful of cases and has been successful.

PAROTIDECTOMY DEFECTS WITH CHEEK SKIN RESECTION

Parotidectomy combined with cheek skin resection is indicated for parotid neoplasms extending to the dermis or through the skin and for preauricular cutaneous malignancy with potential parotid metastasis. In such situations, the first priority is to reconstruct the cheek skin defect and the second priority to fill the missing volume defect (Fig. 4). In many instances when the cheek skin defect is small and the patient has adequate laxity of the cheek and neck skin, elevation followed by primary closure can be performed. Local advancement rotation flaps can also be used for smaller

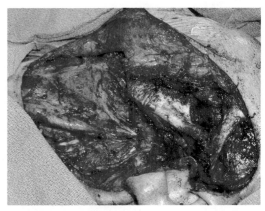

Fig. 4. Large left cheek and temporal skin defect with radical parotidectomy and resection of the masseter muscle.

cheek skin defects. Cervicofacial advancement flaps can also be an option, but this requires fore planning with the ablative team in terms of the skin incisions in the neck. The main advantage of the cervicofacial flaps over free tissue transfer is a better color match to the native cheek skin.

For larger skin defects where advancement rotation flaps cannot cover the defect, free tissue transfer affords the reconstructive surgeon ample options for skin coverage and volume augmentation. For shallow defects requiring skin coverage, a radial forearm free flap is a great choice. The radial forearm flap is based off the radial artery and its vena comitans. An Allen's test is performed before harvesting the flap to ensure adequate vascular supply to the hand through the ulnar artery. The harvesting technique is relatively straightforward. The medial or lateral antebrachial cutaneous nerves can be harvested with the flap to allow for a sensate flap. The radial forearm flap is shown in **Fig. 5** with its associated neurovascular pedicle.

There are several advantages to the radial forearm free flap. It is a thin, pliable skin and fascial flap. These characteristics greatly facilitate contouring the flap over the cheek. For deeper defects, the skin flap can be deepithelialized and tucked onto itself to fill the tissue void. Another advantage is the long pedicle, which can be advantageous in situations in which the superficial temporal vessels are not available. In such cases, the long pedicle can reach the facial vessels in the neck. Generally, a 60 to 70 cm^2 skin paddle area can be harvested from the forearm of an average sized person. In extremely overweight persons,

this flap may have a significant amount of associated subcutaneous tissue necessitating a revision procedure in the future to trim the subcutaneous fat. The radial forearm flap is useful for shallow cheek skin defects.

Larger skin surface area defects require a different type of free flap. The anterolateral thigh free flap offers a larger surface area than the radial forearm. Unlike the radial forearm free flap, the donor site of the anterolateral thigh free flap can be closed primarily without the need for a skin graft. The anterolateral thigh free flap is based off the septocutaneous or musculocutaneous branches off the descending branch of the lateral circumflex femoral artery and vena comitans. The skin perforator is examined by Doppler imaging starting at the midway point between a line drawn from the superior anterior iliac crest to the lateral patella. The skin paddle is centered at the perforator. Generally, an 8-cm wide paddle can be closed primarily. The anatomy of the perforators and the descending circumflex femoral vessels can be variable from patient to patient, making this flap more difficult to harvest than the radial forearm free flap. It can be harvested as a perforator flap or taken with a cuff of vastus lateralis muscle. The associated muscle cuff serves to protect the musculocutaneous perforator and provides additional bulk to fill a three-dimensional tissue defect. In cases not requiring skin reconstruction but with a large tissue defect, the anterolateral thigh skin paddle can be deepithelialized and placed beneath the skin flaps (**Fig. 6**).

For even larger skin defects, the rectus musculocutaneous free flap can be used. This flap is

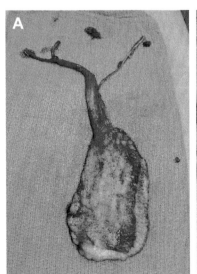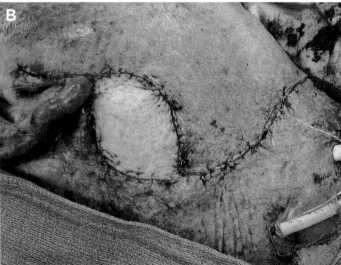

Fig. 5. (*A*) Radial forearm free flap partially deepithelialized from harvesting a split-thickness skin graft to be used for coverage of the donor radial forearm donor site. (*B*) Postoperative appearance with skin paddle showing.

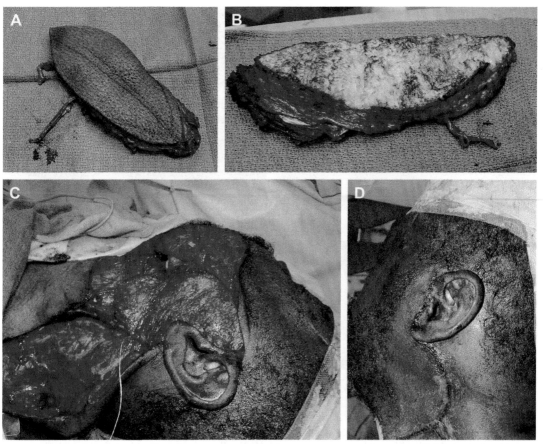

Fig. 6. (A) Anterolateral thigh free flap before deepithelialization. (B) After deepithelialization. (C) Flap inset over the wound. (D) Appearance after skin closure.

especially helpful when parotidectomy is associated with a maxillectomy, orbital exenteration, or infratemporal fossa resection. The rectus muscle provides ample tissue to fill the defect volume, and a larger skin paddle size can be obtained than with the anterolateral thigh flap. The rectus musculocutaneous free flap is based on the inferior epigastric artery and vena comitans. Generally, the preumbilical area has the highest density of musculocutaneous perforators, and this is the area where the skin paddle is harvested (Fig. 7). Another advantage of the rectus musculocutaneous flap is that it can be harvested with two skin paddles for cases in which buccal mucosa is resected. The two main limitations in terms of its utility for parotidectomy defect reconstruction are the limited pedicle length and patient body habitus. Patients who are obese or who have a large pannus usually have a thick subcutaneous layer which limits the use of the skin paddle. In such cases, a rectus muscle free flap can be used to fill the volume defect, and a cervicofacial advancement rotation flap can be used to close the skin. A skin graft can be applied to the rectus

muscle, but this is not as cosmetically favorable as a skin paddle. The anterior rectus sheath defect is usually closed primarily. When a large defect exists, synthetic mesh or AlloDerm can be used to reinforce the anterior rectus sheath.

FACIAL NERVE

The facial nerve is of prime importance during any parotid surgery. The main morbidity of parotid surgery depends on the status of the facial nerve or its branches. Temporary weakness is expected when the nerve is manipulated during the procedure or from heat transfer. If the main trunk of the facial nerve or one of its branches is severed either accidentally or due to tumor involvement, permanent paralysis will ensue. If the facial nerve is transected for tumor infiltration, the reconstructive surgeon must ensure clear margins by frozen section. At this point, facial nerve grafting will need to be performed. Generally, the great auricular nerve on the ipsilateral or contralateral neck is sufficient to cable graft from the main trunk to either upper or lower divisions. Occasionally, the great auricular nerve may

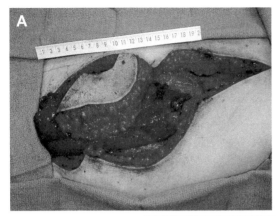
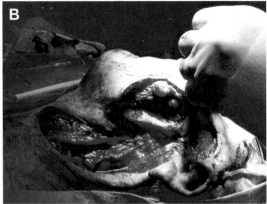
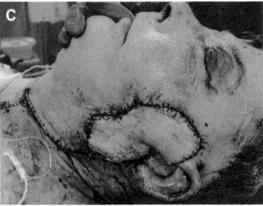

Fig. 7. (A) Rectus abdominus free flap before transfer to the head and neck. (B) The composite defect of the pre-auricular region and neck with skin loss is demonstrated. (C) The flap has been inset into the wound. The muscle and subcutaneous tissue bulks up the tissue loss and the skin allows closure of the wound.

have a branch long enough to anastamose to the zygomatic and marginal mandibular distal branches. More often than not, if the upper and lower divisions need to grafted, the sural nerve or lateral antebrachial cutaneous nerves need to be harvested. The neurorrhaphy is performed using 9-0 nylon suture through the epineureum of the nerve segments. Usually, two to four sutures are placed depending on the size of the nerve.

Additional procedures for facial reanimation need to be addressed either at the time of the ablative procedure or postoperatively depending on the expected outcome. If the upper division or the main trunk is transected, the patient will be expected to have postoperative lagophthalmos; therefore, many reconstructive surgeons will place a 1.2-g gold weight in the affected upper lid. This procedure is reversible if the facial nerve function returns after several months. In addition to the gold weight implant, an inferior lid tarsal strip procedure is performed to prevent ectropion of the lower eyelid. Additional facial reanimation procedures to address the lower lip droop and the nasal valve collapse can be performed at the time of the ablative procedure

or at a later date. These additional procedures are discussed more fully elsewhere in this issue.

SUMMARY

Parotidectomy defects range from small defects to much larger defects including other surrounding tissues. From a reconstructive view, placing autogenous tissue between the parotid bed and the skin flap decreases the incidence of Frey's syndrome and improves the postoperative cosmetic appearance. There are a variety of reconstructive options, and the choice of the most appropriate depends on the patient's wishes, the size of the defect accounting for surface area, and the defect volume. Special attention should also be given to facial nerve rehabilitation.

REFERENCES

1. Berard M. Etirpation de a Parotide. Memoires Observations Extaits 1823;2:60–6.
2. Govindaraj S, et al. The use of acellular dermis in the prevention of Frey's syndrome. Laryngoscope 2001;111: 1993–8.

3. Curry JM, et al. Superficial musculoaponeurotic system elevation and fat graft reconstruction after superficial parotidectomy. Laryngoscope 2008;118: 210–5.

4. Jost G, Legent F, Blaupelot S. Le Comblement des Depressions Residuelle Apres Parotidectomie par un Lambeua de Sterno-cleido-mastoidien. Ann Otol Laryng 1968;85:357–60.

5. Casler JD, Conley J. Sternocleidomastoid muscle transfer and superficial musculoaponeurotic system plication in the prevention of Frey's syndrome. Laryngoscope 1991;101:95–100.

Facial Transplantation: The Next Frontier in Head and Neck Reconstruction

Eunice E. Park, MD, MPH[a], Eric M. Genden, MD[a,b,c],*

KEYWORDS

- Reconstruction • Microvascular • Face
- Transplant • Surgery

Facial reconstruction of extensive defects poses a unique surgical challenge that must take into account the skin color, texture, and complex movement associated with facial expression. Failure to account for these considerations can be dehumanizing. More challenging and equally important are the functional aspects of the face that often are compromised after trauma, burn injury, or surgical resection. The functional consequences of incomplete restoration of the eyelids and the lips can lead to blindness and oral incompetence.

Conventional approaches to facial reconstruction are largely dictated by the extent of the defect. Although smaller defects may be amenable to local flaps, more extensive defects often require free tissue transfer or split-thickness skin grafts. These techniques may suffice to provide coverage; however, they fail to provide a color or texture match and, more importantly, are unable to restore function and movement. Microvascular free flap reconstruction has played an important role in providing coverage for extensive defects that otherwise may represent a risk for infection; however, the cosmetic and functional results are suboptimal. More importantly, microvascular free tissue transfer is a technique that has opened the door to considering the role of microvascular

allotransplantation for the management of extensive facial defects.

Composite tissue allotransplantation (CTA) refers to the transplantation of a heterogeneous group of tissues, including skin, muscle, nerve, and, in some cases, bone. Unlike solid organ transplantation, CTA involves the transplantation of a variety of different tissues each with its own unique antigenic profile. As a result, immunosuppression to prevent rejection can be complex and not always achievable for prolonged periods without leading to systemic toxicity. Skin-bearing transplants are particularly unique because of the high level of antigen-presenting cells residing within the dermis. To prevent rejection, high doses of immunosuppression often are required. Such high levels of immunosuppression are associated with acute and chronic toxicities. Earlier experiences and lessons learned from hand transplants performed in France, China, and Louisville, Kentucky, highlight the multifaceted and complex nature of maintaining a successful transplant.[1] Failure to comply with the immunosuppressive regimen, as demonstrated by the hand transplantation experience, inevitably leads to rejection and graft loss.

The issues surrounding the ethics and science of facial transplantation are interesting and

[a] Department of Otolaryngology-Head and Neck Surgery, The Mount Sinai Medical Center, 1 Gustave L. Levy Place, Box 1189, New York, NY 10029, USA
[b] Institute for Immunobiology, The Mount Sinai Medical Center, 1 Gustave L. Levy Place, Box 1189, New York, NY 10029, USA
[c] Head and Neck Cancer Center, The Mount Sinai Medical Center, 1 Gustave L. Levy Place, Box 1189, New York, NY 10029, USA
* Corresponding author. The Mount Sinai Medical Center, 1 Gustave L. Levy Place, Box 1189, New York, NY 10029.
E-mail address: Eric.Genden@mountsinai.org (E.M. Genden).

Facial Plast Surg Clin N Am 17 (2009) 271–277
doi:10.1016/j.fsc.2009.01.007
1064-7406/09/$ – see front matter © 2009 Elsevier Inc. All rights reserved.

controversial. As transplant immunology is understood better, the potential applications are limitless. Although the ethics of such programs are actively debated, the role of microsurgery in achieving such transplantations is essential.

HISTORY

Early experiences with CTA involved hand transplants, first performed in Lyon, France, and Louisville, Kentucky, in 1998. The recipient of the first "successful" hand transplant, which recently underwent amputation because of rejection, stated that he experienced pain and burning sensations with no normal sensation in the hand.[1] The patient also became emotionally detached from the allograft and could not incorporate it into his own identity. Further reports from China, in which approximately a dozen unilateral and bilateral hand transplants were performed, revealed that most cases have undergone chronic rejection with progressive loss of function resulting from lack of compliance with immunosuppressive medications and consistent medical follow-up. At least two patients underwent amputation of their transplanted hands.[2] Despite the challenges faced in the area of hand transplants, interest in facial transplantation continues to grow.

In December 2002, at a meeting of the British Association of Plastic, Reconstructive and Esthetic Surgeons, British surgeon Peter Butler announced his intention to perform facial transplantation. This ignited widespread public interest and debate over the implications of facial transplantation. In November 2003, reports from a working party of the British Royal College of Surgeons and the French National Consultative Ethics Committee for Health and Life Sciences concluded that the risks outweighed any perceived benefits and that performing facial transplantation was considered highly experimental until more research was conducted and the rate of complications improved.[3,4] In October 2004, Maria Siemionow and colleagues[4] at the Cleveland Clinic obtained institutional review board approval for facial transplantation in humans.

The first partial face transplant was performed in November 2005. A woman was traumatized by a severe dog bite that resulted in amputation of portions of her middle and lower face (**Fig.** 1A). A team of surgeons in Lyon, France, led by Jean-Michel Dubernard, transplanted the allograft, which included skin, facial muscles, vessels, and nerves.[5] The immediate postoperative course was uneventful. During the third week, mild clinical signs of rejection were encountered and controlled with boluses of steroids. Semmes-Weinstein testing revealed sensory recovery by the 14th postoperative week and at 4 months post surgery the patient had an acceptable aesthetic result (see **Fig.** 1B). Motor recovery followed with improved facial movement at 18 months. A follow-up report deemed the operation a success with respect to function, aesthetic appearance, and psychologic acceptance by the patient.[6]

To date, three partial face transplantations have been performed worldwide. A second case of partial face transplantation was reported in China of a 30-year old man who had been severely injured in a bear attack (**Fig.** 2A). After several unsuccessful reconstruction attempts, the patient underwent CTA. In the postoperative period, the patient had three acute rejection episodes and hyperglycemia, which were managed by an adjustment in immunosuppression protocol, pulsed steroid therapy, and insulin therapy. After transplantation, the patient underwent adjunctive reconstructive procedures to improve his appearance (see **Fig.** 2B). At 2 years post transplantation, the patient had adequate sensory and thermal discrimination but facial nerve function was poor. This was attributed to the severely damaged condition of the recipient's facial nerve despite performing a neural anastomosis.[7] In February 2007, a team led by Laurent Lantieri performed the third transplantation on a 27-year-old man who suffered from neurofibromatosis type 1 (**Fig.** 3A). The patient had a massive plexiform neurofibroma that was infiltrating the central and lower portions of his face resulting in bilateral facial paralysis and severe disfigurement. During transplantation, bilateral arterial, venous, and neural anastomoses were performed. The patient experienced two episodes of acute rejection (days 28 and 64) and cytomegalovirus viremia, which were managed by steroid pulse therapy and intravenous foscarnet.[8] Quantitative sensory testing and electroneuromyographic examination at 12 months showed signs of motor and sensory reinnervation.

Facial transplantation has garnered tremendous interest during recent years, since the first reported case in France in 2005, fueled by reports in the popular media. The controversy over the ethical, immunologic, and psychologic issues, however, remains.

THE ROLE OF MICROSURGERY IN COMPOSITE TISSUE TRANSPLANTATION

Not unlike the sentinel work performed by Taylor demonstrating the vascular territories of candidate donor sites for free tissue transfer to achieve facial transplantation, has it been necessary to

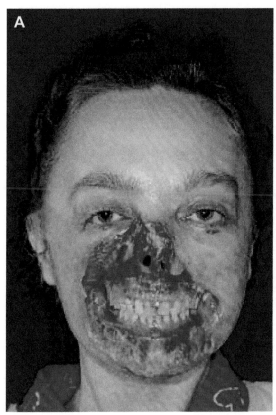
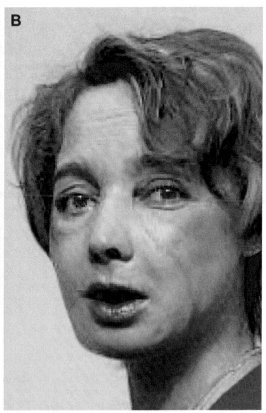

Fig. 1. The first partial face allograft. (*A*) Preoperative image from June 2005. Patient was traumatized after a severe dog bite with amputation of the middle and lower portions of her face. (*B*) Postoperative image 4 months after the first partial face allotransplantation. (*Reprinted from* Devauchelle B, Badet L, Lengelé B, et al. First human face allograft: early report. Lancet 2006;368:204. Copyright [2006]; with permission from Elsevier.)

understand the vascular territories of the face.[9] Early work evaluating the facial vessels demonstrated that although a hemifacial transplant can be performed using the ipsilateral facial artery and vein, a complete facial transplant (**Fig. 4**) requires bilateral facial vessels for revascularization.[10,11] The microsurgical aspects of allotransplantation essentially are the same as those used in free tissue transfer. The viability of the allograft is dependant on the flow through the facial artery and facial vein.[12] Several techniques have been described using the external carotid artery or the facial artery; however, like free tissue transfer, the more blood flow to the flap, the less likely ischemia ensues.

Unique to facial transplantation are the issues of immune-mediated rejection and motor reinnervation. Acute rejection must be prevented at all costs. An early rejection episode may result in acute vascular thrombosis at the site of the microvascular anastomosis or microthombosis in the capillary system located in the distal areas of the

flap. As a result, patients are treated with a strict immunosuppressive regimen that must be maintained for the life of the patient if the graft is to be preserved.[6] Monitoring of the flap perfusion can be accomplished with an external temperature probe, Doppler probe, or skin prick.

Unlike conventional free flap reconstruction, facial transplantation usually requires motor and or sensory reinnervation. Although this is used occasionally for free flap reconstruction of the head and neck, it is commonly used for facial transplantation to provide facial sensation, tone, volitional movement, and oral competence. This requires that a surgeon is comfortable with microneural surgery. An 18-month follow-up after facial transplantation performed by Dubernard and colleagues[6] demonstrated that the patient was able to eat and drink almost normally by the end of the first postoperative week with mild leakage during drinking from her mouth. The oral incompetence had resolved by 12 months. Sensory recovery as assessed by Semmes-Weinstein tests

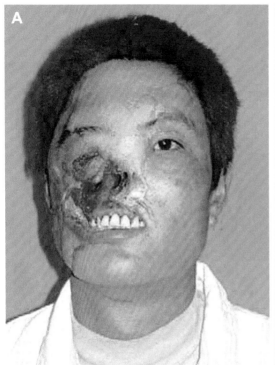 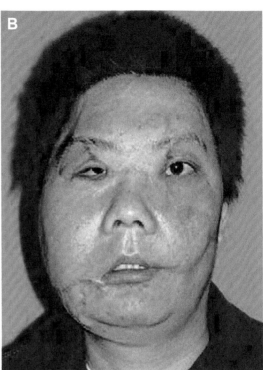

Fig. 2. A partial facial allotransplantation performed in China in 2006. (*A*) A man severely injured in a 2004 bear attack. (*B*) Twenty months post transplantation. (*Reprinted from* Guo S, Han Y, Zhang X, et al. Human facial allotransplantation: a 2-year follow-up study. Lancet 2008;372:632. Copyright [2008]; with permission from Elsevier.)

(light touch sensation studied using static monofilaments) demonstrated that sensory discrimination was recovered and hot and cold sensation nearly normal at 4 months and normal at 6 months over the entire graft.

IMMUNOSUPPRESSION

Unlike other common solid tissue transplants, such as kidney and liver, CTA, like facial transplants, is histologically heterogeneous and contains tissue components that express different antigenic forms. Therefore, allotransplantation mandates substantial lifelong immunosuppression to prevent rejection. Failure of or noncompliance with the regimen could lead to devastating results with the loss of the transplanted face.[13] Unlike most solid organs transplants, which usually are more tolerant of acute rejection, facial CTA is less able to tolerate rejection, and acute rejection may lead to scarring and dysfunction of the graft or fulminate rejection and graft necrosis.[1] Over the past 4 decades, several significant developments in immunosuppression protocol have allowed for long-term survival of partial and complete allotransplanted organs, ranging from 60% to 90% at 5 years depending on the transplanted organ.[14] Achieving

a balance between overimmunosuppression and underimmunosuppression requires an appreciation of other factors, including pretransplant morbidity, pre-existing disease status, nutritional status and post-transplant immunomodulating viral infections.

CTA immunosuppression protocols have been less developed until recently because of the notion that these types of tissue transplants are not essential for survival. Currently, the most commonly used maintenance immunosuppression in kidney transplant recipients in the United States is a tacrolimus, mycophenolate acid, and corticosteroids combination, which also has been successfully used in recent experimental hand and face transplantations.[15] Immunologic risk data, published in 2004 in "Facial Transplantation: A Working Party Report from the Royal College of Surgeons of England,"[16] estimate the likelihood of graft loss at approximately 10% from acute rejection within the first year and of significant loss of graft function from chronic rejection at approximately 30% to 50% of patients over the first 2 to 5 years.[17] To monitor for rejection, Duberand and colleagues[6] used a concomitant radial forearm free flap allograft placed into the submammary fold. This was used as a sentinel

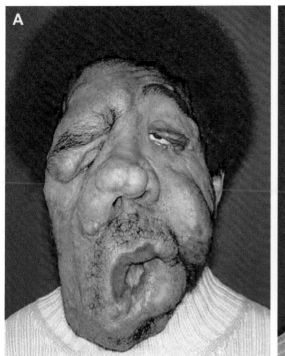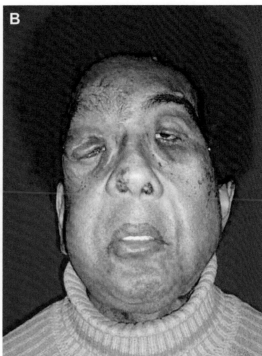

Fig. 3. CTA performed on a patient who had neurofibromatosis type 1. (A) A man who had a massive plexiform neurofibroma infiltrating the central and lower portions of his face. (B) One year post transplantation. (*Reprinted from* Lantieri L, Meningaud JP, Grimbert P, et al. Repair of the lower and middle parts of the face by composite tissue allotransplantation in a patient with massive plexiform neurofibroma: a 1-year follow-up study. Lancet 2008;372:640. Copyright (2008); with permission from Elsevier.)

graft for skin biopsies to limit damage to the grafted face.

ETHICAL CONCERNS

At the center of the ethical debate in facial transplantation is the question, Does potentially improving a patient's quality of life justify the potential long-term risks involved with immunosuppression?[15] The complications of lifelong immunosuppression are well defined and significant side effects, such as increased rates of cancer, infections, and nephrotoxicity, are potentially life-threatening. The etiology of post-transplant malignancy is believed multifactorial in nature and presumably the result of impaired immunosurveillance of neoplastic cells and depressed antiviral immune activity.[18] Recent renal transplant experiences with tacrolimus, mycophenolate mofetil, and steroids combination, which is the current immunosuppressive regimen in CTA, revealed that the cumulative incidence of cancer is lower at the early time point of 3-year follow-up. To date, none of the hand transplant recipients has developed cancer.[15]

The majority of patients who have had a transplant have an infection as a result of immunosuppression. Opportunistic infections include viral infections, fungal infections, and *Pneumocystis carinii* pneumonia. Over the past decade, improved selectivity of immunosuppressive regimens, the availability of new antiviral and antifungal agents, and improved diagnostic accuracy have played a role in decreasing the incidence and severity of post-transplant infections.[17]

As the concept of quality of life for patients has become more important, acceptance of allotransplantation for these less critical transplants has grown significantly. This acceptance has increased as techniques for immunosuppression have become more specific and targeted and have fewer side effects. The ideal immunosuppressive agents target tissue and organ that are transplanted and allow acceptance of the transplanted part without having any other effects on the recipient's tissue. Thus, the ability of a recipient to combat residual cancer or any potential metastatic sites remains intact and this form of targeted immunosuppressant would have no negative effects on the outcomes of the cancer.[14]

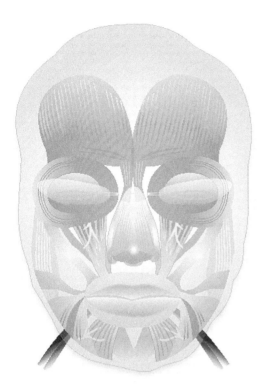

Fig. 4. A complete facial allotransplantation would require bilateral facial vessel and neural anastomoses for revascularization and successful transplantation. (*Courtesy of* Christine C. Kim, Chicago, IL.)

The development of these types of agents will revolutionize microsurgical reconstruction because they would allow transfer of previously unreconstructable, specialized tissues using well-described microsurgical techniques and would maximize the aesthetic and functional results of head and neck reconstruction. The development of highly immunosuppressive agents remains the principal obstacle to taking microsurgical reconstruction to the next level in CTA.[14]

Careful patient selection is critical to the final success of facial transplantation. Failure to comply with the immunosuppressive regimen of medications can have catastrophic results leading to rejection of the facial part. Poor selection of patients could have a negative effect on the future of this reconstructive procedure and fuel ethical and legal disputes. Guiding principles, published by the American Society of Plastic Surgeons and the American Society for Reconstructive Microsurgery, consider facial transplantation an experimental procedure, urging that facial transplantation be attempted only by multidisciplinary teams under institutional review board–approved research protocols.[16] Steps are needed

to balance the risks and benefits of this highly controversial procedure.

FUTURE DIRECTIONS AND CONCLUSION

Although the technical aspects related to microvascular and microneural surgery required to initiate a transplant are well worked out, donor-specific immunotolerance regimens need to be explored further before facial transplantation can be offered to patients routinely. Current immune strategies to achieve tolerance induction include irradiation, donor bone marrow transfusion, intrathymic injection of donor cells, and antibody-based therapies.[1] Future research will be directed in these areas and with progress in nontoxic regimens, there is little question that facial transplantation will play a role in the future of facial reconstruction.

REFERENCES

1. Brenner MJ, Tung TH, Jensen JN, et al. The spectrum of complications of immunosuppression: is the time right for hand transplantation? J Bone Joint Surg Am 2002;84-A(10):1861–70.
2. Okie S. Facial transplantation: brave new face. N Engl J Med 2006;354(9):889–94.
3. Huxtable R, Woodley J. Gaining face or losing face? Framing the debate on face transplants. Bioethics 2005;19(5–6):505–22.
4. Siemionow M, Sonmez E. Face as an organ. Ann Plast Surg 2008;61(3):345–52.
5. Devauchelle B, Badet L, Lengelé B, et al. First human face allograft: early report. Lancet 2006; 368(9531):203–9.
6. Dubernard JM, Lengelé B, Morelon E, et al. Outcomes 18 months after the first human partial face transplantation. N Engl J Med 2007;357(24):2451–60.
7. Guo S, Han Y, Zhang X, et al. Human facial allotransplantation: a 2-year follow-up study. Lancet 2008; 372(9639):631–8.
8. Lantieri L, Meningaud JP, Grimbert P, et al. Repair of the lower and middle parts of the face by composite tissue allotransplantation in a patient with massive plexiform neurofibroma: a 1-year follow-up study. Lancet 2008;372(9639):639–45.
9. Baccarani A, Follmar KE, Baumeister SP, et al. Technical and anatomical considerations of face harvest in face transplantation. Ann Plast Surg 2006;57(5):483–8.
10. Yazici I, Cavusoglu T, Comert A, et al. Maxilla allograft for transplantation: an anatomical study. Ann Plast Surg 2008;61(1):105–13.
11. Wang HY, Li QF, Zheng SW, et al. Cadaveric comparison of two facial flap-harvesting techniques for alloplastic facial transplantation. J Plast Reconstr Aesthet Surg 2007;60(11):1175–81.

12. Kelly M, Butler PE. Patient selection for facial transplantation I: anatomical and surgical considerations. Int J Surg 2004;2(2):114–5 [discussion: 115–6].

13. Warnke PH. Repair of a human face by allotransplantation. Lancet 2006;368(9531):181–3.

14. Cordeiro PG. Frontiers in free flap reconstruction in the head and neck. J Surg Oncol 2008;97(8):669–73.

15. Pomahac B, Aflaki P, Chandraker A, et al. Facial transplantation and immunosuppressed patients: a new frontier in reconstructive surgery. Transplantation 2008;85(12):1693–7.

16. ASRM/ASPS. Facial transplantation—ASRM/ASPS guiding principles. Available at: http://www.microsurg.org/ftGuidelines.pdf. Accessed September 1, 2008.

17. Vasilic D, Alloway RR, Barker JH, et al. Risk assessment of immunosuppressive therapy in facial transplantation. Plast Reconstr Surg 2007;120(3):657–68.

18. Wimmer CD, Rentsch M, Crispin A, et al. The janus face of immunosuppressio—de novo malignancy after renal transplantation: the experience of the Transplantation Center Munich. Kidney Int 2007;71(12):1271–8.

Free Tissue Transfer in the Reconstruction of Massive Skin Cancer

Mark K. Wax, MD, FACS, FRCS(C)

KEYWORDS

• Skin cancer • Reconstruction • Free tissue transfer

Of all the malignancies encountered in the head and neck, skin cancer is by far the most common. It is estimated that one in six Americans will develop skin cancer at some point in their life. The head and neck area sees a disproportionate amount of these cancers because of its predilection to be exposed to the harmful effects of ultraviolet radiation. Compared with other areas of the body, the skin of the head and neck is more often exposed to the sun. Most sun-induced lesions on the skin of the head and neck are benign. Unfortunately, many may be premalignant or malignant. The skin of the head and neck plays an important role in individuals' perceptions of themselves and other people's perceptions of them; thus lesions of the surface area of the skin of the head and neck are easily detectable. Compared with malignancies of the skin in other areas of the body, which may be of a considerable size before they present to medical personnel, most lesions on the human face are detected at an early phase by either the patient or their family.[1] Oftentimes the smallest lesion on the face or neck is notable to patients or an associate of theirs, thus driving the patient to seek medical attention. Most tumors of the skin in the head and neck are best treated by surgical excision. Most lesions can be primarily reconstructed or allowed to heal by secondary intention. Occasionally, recurrent tumors or those that extend deeper than average may require composite tissue resection involving the underlying tissues. In this case, reconstruction is not easily accomplished by local flaps or secondary intention. The composite tissue loss requires composite tissue for reconstruction.

Most skin cancers involve the surface epithelium, only rarely extending into the subcutaneous tissue. Occasionally, patients may present with a neglected tumor, a recurrent tumor, or a fast-growing lesion that involves deeper structures (**Fig. 1**). These tumors may involve the subcutaneous structures, the facial skeleton, or even adjacent organ systems. Treatment usually involves composite modalities with resection of the adjacent tissues followed by postoperative radiotherapy.[1–4] The surgical defect can be devastating from both functional and cosmetic perspectives (**Fig. 2**). Because a significant number of these lesions are secondary to recurrence, the patient may have had multiple surgical excisions in the past. Usually, local flaps have been used several times or the patient may have already undergone radiotherapy. The ability to use local tissue requires movement of tissue from adjacent areas; prior treatment leaves the local tissues unavailable for reconstruction. Before the advent of free tissue transfer, many of these patients would have been rehabilitated with a prosthesis. Although beyond the scope of this article, prosthetic rehabilitation in the hands of a well-trained prosthodontist is an excellent modality for reconstruction. Patient satisfaction with cosmetic and functional outcomes can be exceedingly high. The work involved in maintaining the prosthesis and positioning it so that it does not slip and maintains its proper orientation when the patient is out and about can become burdensome. Cost and availability of skilled prosthodontists further weigh into the equation because these may not be available in the location from which the patient originates (**Fig. 3**).

Department of Otolaryngology-Head and Neck Surgery, Oregon Health & Science University, Physicians Pavilion 2nd Floor, 3181 SW Sam Jackson Park Road PV-01, Portland, OR 97239-3098, USA
E-mail address: waxm@ohsu.edu

Facial Plast Surg Clin N Am 17 (2009) 279–286
doi:10.1016/j.fsc.2009.01.009
1064-7406/09/$ – see front matter

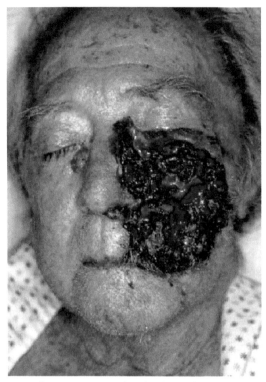

Fig. 1. This man presented with a large skin cancer that had been present for a long time. He had refused treatment for many years.

Introduction of free tissue transfer into the reconstructive paradigm for head and neck cancer allowed the reconstructive surgeon to replace composite tissue loss with composite tissue. The ability to replace complex tissue structures, such as the mandible with its overlying skin or mucosal covering, with composite bone mucosal vascularized tissue was shown to drastically reduce the morbidity encountered in patients. Functional rehabilitation and cosmetic outcomes were also demonstrated to be markedly superior to previous reconstructive methodologies.[5] This reconstructive paradigm has been directly translated into that for patients who have massive skin cancers. Resection of these lesions often entails removal of cutaneous tissue, subcutaneous bone, and various organ systems. Free tissue transfer allows one to tailor the reconstructive material to replace these composite defects with similar tissue characteristics. The ability to tailor the volume of tissue transferred specific to the volume of tissue resected allows for a much better cosmetic outcome (**Fig. 4**). Recently, reinnervation with sensory nerves has allowed for the theoretic development of sensation of the resected area with the free tissue transfer. Whether this is beneficial has not been determined.

Most tumors involving the skin of the head and neck are easily treated by local resection and reconstruction. Facial plastic and reconstructive surgeons over the years have devised multiple local and regional flaps that allow for excellent cosmetic and functional outcomes. These reconstructive options have ranged from no intervention (letting the wound granulate) to multiple and often ingenious rotation advancement and other types of local flaps. Reconstruction of the composite tissue defects involving the lower eyelid or the nasal bone and cartilage can often be repaired using combinations of turn-in flaps, cartilage harvested from other areas, and local rotation flaps or forehead-type flaps. Overall, the cosmetic and functional results are excellent. There is a subgroup of patients who have undergone previous treatments for their head and neck skin cancers. These may include surgical resection with flap reconstruction and often include radiation therapy. It is this subgroup of patients who have had multiple treatment modalities over a prolonged period of time who present unique reconstructive problems. Our patient population has demonstrated that 50% of patients who have massive cutaneous carcinomas have more than six previous attempts at cure. Radiotherapy is often one of those attempts.

Overall, one must be aware that free tissue transfer is a last resort for skin cancer of the head and neck. One of the largest series in the literature involved 43 patients who required free tissue transfer for reconstruction of their defects.[1] This series has since been updated to 87. Patients requiring free tissue transfer can be divided into two groups based on the cause. The first group is those patients who present with large fungating lesions often involving cartilaginous or bony structures. We have labeled this group as the massively neglected skin cancers because these tumors are often present for many years. They are slow growing and follow the natural course of a malignancy with local invasion and destruction of the surrounding tissues (**Fig 5**). They are an average 10 to 15 cm in size, fungating, and often infected. The prime factor in their development has been patient denial and thus many ingenious methods of covering the tumor have been devised by the patient to avoid medical care. Often the family is aware of the tumor but conceded to the patient's wishes; only when extraneous forces, such as neighbors, police, or other individuals, are present does the patient seek medical help. These tumors rarely present with metastatic disease. When they are treated, local control is the main goal.

The second group of patients are those who have been heavily pretreated in the past. Although

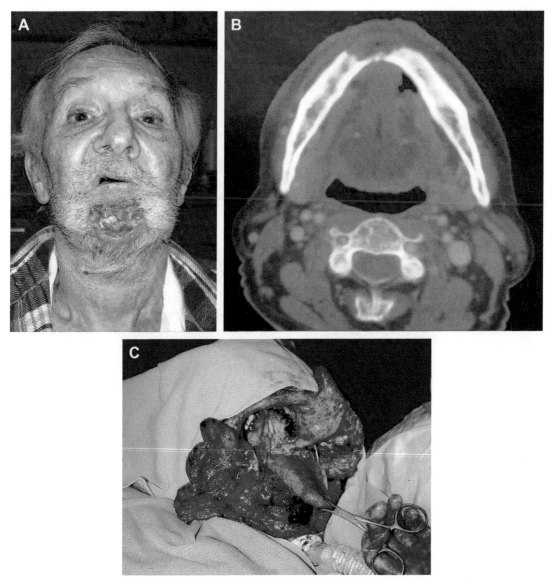

Fig. 2. (*A*) This man presented with a large neglected basal cell cancer of the chin. (*B*) Panographic examination reveals destruction of the underlying bone. (*C*) Surgical excision leaves a composite defect involving mandible, floor of mouth, and the chin.

the first group has mainly basal cell carcinoma, this group has a combination of basal or squamous cell carcinomas that have recurred multiple times. More than half of these patients have undergone between one and five treatments, whereas the other half have undergone six or more treatments. Most of these patients have undergone radiation therapy as one of their treatment modalities. Almost all of these patients have had some form of reconstructive procedure during one of their excisions. The treatment of the recurrent tumor often entails not only adequate resection of the local tissue but also resection of the

reconstructed area with its accompanying flap and other contiguous structures. The local tissues are then not amenable to local rotation advancement because underlying scarring from previous dissection or from radiation therapy has made that option untenable. Because these tumors often involve deeper subcutaneous structures or other composite tissues, such as the orbital contents, the oracle, nose, mandible, maxilla, or lateral temporal bone, tissue volumes are such that local rotation advancement flaps do not provide an adequate reconstructive option. The volume and need for healthy tissue require free tissue transfer.

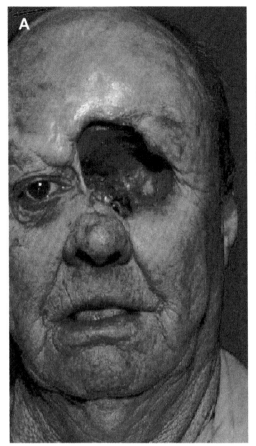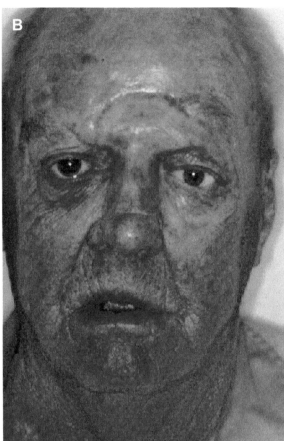

Fig. 3. (*A*) This gentleman underwent a large composite resection for a recurrent skin cancer. (*B*) The resulting defect was rehabilitated with a prosthesis, which he rarely wore.

Our series of 87 patients revealed that the histology was similar between the two groups of patients. Other underlying factors other than neglect in the one group and multiple treatments in the second group were equal between groups. The tissues that required resection were often similar between the two groups. Not only was there a large soft tissue cutaneous defect, but other ablative procedures and contiguous structures were resected as required. As can be seen from **Table 1** the defect was indeed large, deep, and complex with either the orbit or maxilla removed in many cases. The other issue in this region is that often the tumor has spread beyond the craniofacial skeleton so that cranial bone is resected or a craniofacial resection is required. In these cases separation of the intracranial contents from the outside is necessary. Pericranial flaps, the mainstay of reconstruction in the untreated patient, are not applicable in these pretreated or massive lesions.

Most tumors that require free tissue transfer reconstruction originate on the cheek, with the next most common location being fairly evenly split between the ear, nose, forehead, and scalp. The orbit was frequently involved with it being difficult to tell if the primary tumor originated from the cheek or the eyelids. **Table 2** demonstrates the originating site of the tumor; this is similar to the location of primary skin cancers that require local resection in the head and neck area.

The primary advantage for free tissue transfer is that it allows reconstruction of composite tissue with similar composite tissue. Other articles in this issue deal with the specific subsites of the scalp and forehead, lip, midface, lateral temporal bone, parotid, and the orbit and orbital exenteration. In general, the oncologic surgeon is usually able to predict the defect so that the ablative surgeon could predict both the volume of tissue and the composite nature of the tissue that will be required for the reconstruction.[6,7] As one would predict, the defect is often larger than expected due to retraction of the tissues after incision and resection.

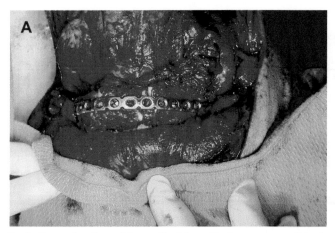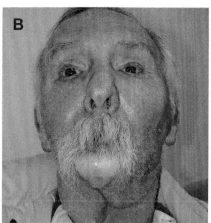

Fig. 4. Reconstruction of the patient from **Fig. 1** was accomplished with a fibular free tissue transfer. (*A*) A fibula has been used to reconstruct the mandible. (*B*) Postoperative cosmesis and function are acceptable.

This inelasticity of the remaining tissues mandates that the reconstructive surgeon be ready to reconstruct a larger defect (**Fig. 6**). Choice of flap must also take into account the three-dimensional structure of the defect. A large "divot" with large surface area may require the bulk and ability to fill nooks and crannies with muscle. Another large surface area may require an anterolateral thigh flap when the depth is not too great.

Before one undertakes a resection with reconstruction in patients who have such large and extensive tumors, prognosis in survival and local control should be taken into consideration. The oncologic ablation often involves multiple composite structures. The demands on resources for the patient, hospital, and the surgical staff can be considerable. As in other head and neck oncologic processes, before one embarks on a treatment regimen that may involve maxillectomy, craniofacial resection, or orbital exenteration with a free flap reconstruction, we must be sure that our treatment and our rehabilitation will allow for a reasonable quality of life with local regional control. There is not much in the literature concerning the long-term prognosis and survival in patients who have massive skin cancers. Most reports are single institutional studies that often have low numbers or are small case reports. Our series has evaluated 87 patients treated over a 17-year period. We have found that survival was acceptable with 55% of patients obtaining local regional control. Perineural invasion seemed to be a prognostic indicator when evaluated through univariant analysis.

Fig. 7 demonstrates that the ability to attain local regional control depends highly on whether there is perineural invasion present in a main nerve. Forty percent of patients who have perineural invasion end up with positive margins in the nerve. If one looks at the overall group, 40% of patients end up with some form of positive margin. In the vast majority of these patients, it will be due to perineural invasion of a named nerve. Because the most common site of tumor is in the cheek or eyelids, V1 and V2 are the most common nerves involved in perineural extension, often with extension along the nerve through the skull base. When these cancers recur locally it is often deep in the wound at the skull base junction. The involvement of the skull base or intracranial spread makes them difficult to re-treat. Direct invasion of the facial nerve was rarely seen unless there was metastatic disease into the lymph nodes with extracapsular spread or invasion by a skin cancer into the parotid. The ability to obtain clear margins is the strongest prognostic indicator for these tumors. Although

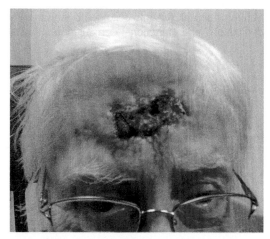

Fig. 5. This woman has had forehead skin cancer for many years. It was suggested that she have it removed but she has refused.

Table 1
Structures removed during the surgical resection

Structure	Patient no.
Orbital contents	29
Maxilla	22
Mandible	7
Auricle	9
Craniofacial resection	17
Nasal structure	6
Lateral temporal bone	13

not affected by histology or the underlying presentation (be it massive neglected tumor or previous multiple treatments), perineural invasion demonstrates a local regional recurrence rate of almost 80% with only a 20% survival rate. If the margins are negative, then roughly 90% of patients survive at 5 years. Our policy has been to treat all these patients with Mohs micrographic surgery or frozen section analysis of the peripheral margins and the deep margin to evaluate their status. If they have not had previous radiation, patients often should be given radiation postoperatively. Patients who have had previous radiation are often candidates for further radiation. The resection of the tumor and the underlying tissue removes all the tissue that has seen the previous radiation. The free tissue transfer that has been used to reconstruct the defect will tolerate a course of radiation.[8]

Functional reconstruction can be obtained with excellent results. The ability to use free tissue transfer to separate the oral cavity and the nasal cavity or nasopharynx is easily and consistently performed. No patient in our series required an obturator and all patients obtained adequate oral deglutition and functional articulation. Dental rehabilitation is often not possible in this patient population, but most of these patients do not use dental rehabilitation before their surgery. Most patients are able to eat and drink well. Deglutition with dysphagia is only affected if significant oral cavity or oropharyngeal mucosa or neural structures are involved and resected. The ability to permanently separate the cranial contents from the oral or nasal cavity is successful.[8]

Cosmetic outcomes when defects are deep and laterally based are usually excellent. When patients have orbital exenterations or large resections involving composite structures of the maxilla or nasal cavity, then the cosmetic outcome is marginal. Although rehabilitation and ability to be out in public are often possible, surgical reconstruction of normal structures can be more difficult.

Overall, the functional and cosmetic outcomes would enforce the principle that these tumors are worth treating. Survival rates in patients who have perineural invasion are poor and further investigation to be able to delineate this subpatient population needs to be done. If ancillary or adjuvant treatments can be instituted they certainly should be used in all patients.

Table 2
Site of origin of the primary tumor

Site	Patient no.
Cheek/eyelids	31
Parotid/lateral temporal bone	14
Scalp	14
Ear	9
Nose	8
Forehead	7
Neck	4

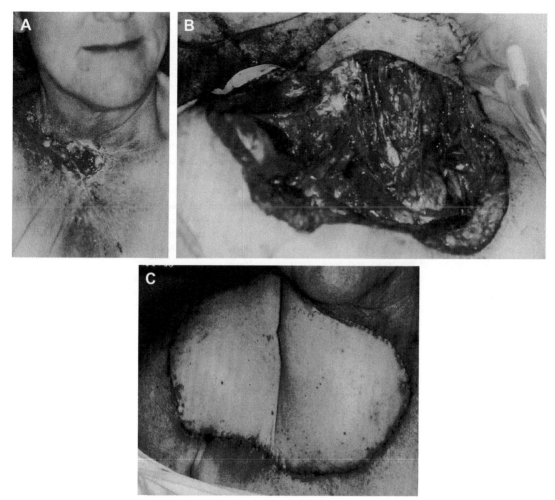

Fig. 6. (A) This woman has a neglected and previously treated basal cell carcinoma of the skin of the neck. (B) After resection, a large soft tissue defect of considerable surface area is left. (C) The defect has been reconstructed with a large composite free rectus abdominus flap.

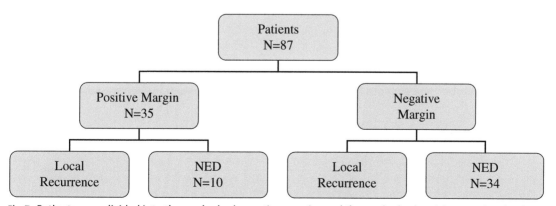

Fig. 7. Patients were divided into those who had negative margins and those who had positive margins, (perineural or microscopic). Survival and recurrence were related to margin status.

SUMMARY

Skin cancer arising in the head and neck is a common occurrence. Although the vast majority of these can be treated with simple excision and local reconstruction there is a subset of patients who have massive tumors that require composite tissue resection. These patients are best reconstructed with free tissue transfer. Acceptable functional and cosmetic results can be expected. Long-term survival is excellent in patients who have negative margins.

REFERENCES

1. Wax MK, Burkey BB, Bascom D, et al. The role of free tissue transfer in the reconstruction of massive neglected skin cancers of the head and neck. Arch Facial Plast Surg 2003;5:479–83.
2. Levine H. Cutaneous carcinoma of the head and neck: management of massive and previously uncontrolled lesions. Laryngoscope 1983;93:87–105.
3. Dias FL, Sa GM, Kligerman J, et al. Prognostic factors and outcome in craniofacial surgery for malignant cutaneous tumors involving the anterior skull base. Arch Otolaryngol Head Neck Surg 1997;123:738–42.
4. Ahn ST, Hruza GJ, Mustoe TA. Microvascular free tissue reconstruction following Mohs' micrographic surgery for advanced head and neck skin cancer. Head Neck 1991;13:145–52.
5. Wax MK, Rosenthal EL, Winslow CP, et al. The ulnar fasciocutaneous free flap in head and neck reconstruction. Laryngoscope 2002;112(12):2155–60.
6. Lutz BS, Wei FC, Chen HC, et al. Reconstruction of scalp defects with free flaps in 30 cases. Br J Plast Surg 1998;51:186–90.
7. Beasley NJ, Gilbert RW, Gullane PJ, et al. Scalp and forehead reconstruction using free revascularized tissue transfer. Arch Facial Plast Surg 2004;6(1): 16–20.
8. Funk GF, Laurenzo JF, Valentino J, et al. Free tissue transfer reconstruction of midfacial and cranio-orbito-facial defects. Arch Otolaryngol Head Neck Surg 1995;121:293–303.

Erratum
New Concepts in Nasal Tip Contouring

Dean M. Toriumi, MD, Mark A. Checcone, MD

This article appeared in the February 2009 issue of the *Facial Plastic Surgery Clinics of North America* (Volume 17, Number 1). The credit lines were omitted from several figures. The proper credit lines for these figures are as follows:

Figs. 4, 5, 6, 8, 9, 10, 11, 12, 13, 14, 15, 18, 19, 20, 21, 22, 24, 27, 28, 29, 30, 31, 33, 34, 35, 36, 37, and 38:
From Toriumi DM. New concepts in nasal tip contouring. Arch Facial Plast Surg 2006;8:156–85; with permission. Copyright © 2006, American Medical Association. All rights reserved.

Fig. 16A:
From Toriumi DM. Structure approach in rhinoplasty. Facial Plast Surg Clin North Am 2002;10:1–22; with permission.

Figs. 16B and 17:
From Toriumi DM. Structural approach to primary rhinoplasty. Aesthet Surg J 2002;22:72–84; with permission.

Fig. 23:
From Toriumi DM, Patel AB, DeRosa J. Correcting the short nose in revision rhinoplasty. Facial Plast Surg Clin North Am 2006;14:343–55; with permission.

Fig. 26:
From DeRosa, J, Toriumi, DM. Toriumi approach. In: Gunter JP, Rohrich RJ, Adams WP, editors. Dallas rhinoplasty: nasal surgery by the masters. 2nd edition. St. Louis: Quality Medical Publishing; 2007. p. 1391–420; with permission.

Facial Plast Surg Clin N Am 17 (2009) 287
doi:10.1016/j.fsc.2009.04.001
1064-7406/09/$ – see front matter © 2009 Elsevier Inc. All rights reserved.

Index

Note: Page numbers of article titles are in **boldface** type.

A

Adipose tissue. See *Fat entries.*
Adjunctive techniques, in periauricular and temporal
    bone defect reconstruction, 258–259
    in scalp reconstruction, 186–187
    radiotherapy as. See *Radiation therapy.*
Advancement flaps, cervicofacial, in orbital complex
    reconstruction, 228–229
        in parotid defect reconstruction, 266
    in major lip defect reconstruction, 204
    in massive skin cancer reconstruction, 281
    in maxillofacial trauma reconstruction, 242
    in parotid defect reconstruction, 265–266
    in scalp reconstruction, 184–185
    in total nasal defect reconstruction, 198
Aerodigestive tract, in orbital complex
    reconstruction, 225
Aesthetic goals, for reconstruction. See *Cosmesis.*
Airway, nasal, functional anatomy of, 192
        in periauricular and temporal bone defect
            reconstruction, 259
    stabilization, for maxillofacial trauma
        reconstruction, 240
Allogeneic barrier, in parotid defect reconstruction,
    263
Alloplastic reconstruction, of scalp, 187
Allotransplantation, in facial transplantation. See
    Composite tissue allotransplantation (CTA).
Alopecia, scalp reconstruction and, 178–179, 181,
    183–185
Ancillary procedures. See *Adjunctive techniques.*
Anterolateral thigh (ALT) free flap, in major lip defect
    reconstruction, 204–207
    in massive skin cancer reconstruction, 283
    in orbital complex reconstruction, 227
    in parotid defect reconstruction, 266–267
    in periauricular and temporal bone defect
        reconstruction, 257–258
Aramany classification, of midface and maxilla
    defects, 212–213
Arteries. See *Vascular structures.*
Asymmetry. See *Facial contour asymmetry.*
Auricular nerve, in parotid defect reconstruction,
    267–268
    in periauricular and temporal bone defect
        reconstruction, 258–259
Auricular reconstruction, in periauricular and
    temporal bone defect reconstruction, 259

Autogenic barrier, in parotid defect reconstruction, 263
Autografts, in scalp reconstruction, 187
Avulsive trauma, to face, maxillofacial reconstruction
    for, 240–250

B

Bacterial count, in necrotic tissue, of maxillofacial
    trauma, 241
Ballistic trauma, to face, maxillofacial trauma
    reconstruction for, 240–250
Basal cell carcinoma, massive head and neck
    reconstruction for, 281, 285
    of skull base, 253
    orbital complex reconstruction for, microvascular,
        231–234
    scalp reconstruction for, chronic nonhealing
        wound with, 180–181
        Moh's excision and, 179–180
Biologic creep, with tissue expansion, in scalp
    reconstruction, 181–183
Blunt trauma, to face, maxillofacial reconstruction for,
    240
Bone anatomy, of nose, 192
Bone defects, massive skin cancer reconstruction
    and, 280–282
    periauricular and temporal, reconstruction of,
        253–262. See also *Periauricular bone defects;*
        Temporal bone defects.
Bone exposure, with periauricular and temporal bone
    defect reconstruction, 260
Bone grafts, calvarial, in orbital complex
    reconstruction, 234–236
    in maxillofacial trauma reconstruction, 243, 249
        cranial, 241–242, 246
        free, 246
        mandibular, 243–244
        maxillary, 242, 246
        nasal, 247–248
    in scalp reconstruction, 187
    in total nasal defect reconstruction, 196
    vascularized, in major lip defect reconstruction,
        205, 207
        in maxillofacial trauma reconstruction,
            243–244
        in midface and maxilla reconstruction,
            219–221
        in orbital complex reconstruction, 225–228,
            231, 234–235

facialplastic.theclinics.com

Moving?

Make sure your subscription moves with you!

To notify us of your new address, find your **Clinics Account Number** (located on your mailing label above your name), and contact customer service at:

E-mail: elspcs@elsevier.com

800-654-2452 (subscribers in the U.S. & Canada)
314-453-7041 (subscribers outside of the U.S. & Canada)

Fax number: 314-523-5170

Elsevier Periodicals Customer Service
11830 Westline Industrial Drive
St. Louis, MO 63146

*To ensure uninterrupted delivery of your subscription, please notify us at least 4 weeks in advance of move.